Kind Hearts

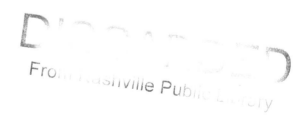

Kind Hearts

Self-Esteem and the Challenges of Aging

by James Frush, Ph.D.

Starrhill Press
Montgomery

Library of Congress Cataloging-in-Publication Data:
Frush, James.
Kind hearts : self-esteem and the challenges of aging /
by James Frush.
p. cm.
Includes bibliographical references and index.
ISBN 1-57359-036-3
1. Self-esteem in old age. I. Title.
BF724.85.S39 F78 2000
155.67'182--dc21
00-011022

Designed by Lissa Monroe and Jim Davis.

Printed in the United States.

Starrhill Press, an imprint of Black Belt Publishing, LLC, publishes high-quality nonfiction books on a variety of topics including art, gardening, health, history, literature, music, and travel. We also publish the popular Starrhill Calendar. The imprint began in 1983.

Dedication

To my wife, Carol, and our children Michael, Gloria, and Gus, who have given my life love and richness. To my mother, whose nurturing eclipsed the most archetypal of Jewish mothers. To my father, whose patience, confidence, and love never wavered.

Contents

Acknowledgments

This book owes much to a number of people:

I thank Pam McCreary, who typed the first draft of the manuscript, and most especially Mary Ann Logan, who typed the seemingly endless revisions of the final draft.

I thank my friend Dr. James White for his encouragement, editorial suggestions, and guidance.

I thank my editor, Jim Davis, and the owners and staff of Starrhill Press.

Finally, I thank the many heart attack survivors I have interviewed during the past twelve years, and the hundreds of elderly persons I have talked with and learned from over the past thirty-five years. Each of them holds a special place in my heart.

Introduction

To this day, when I go to my favorite restaurant in Marin County, California, I stare momentarily at one of the booths adjacent to the counter. It is the booth my father and I sat in on the day he told me that he was going to die within the next four years.

Before we had lunch, he had seen his doctor. The doctor confirmed what a friend, an internist who lived out of town, suspected. Months before, Dad had experienced a "silent" coronary, a type of coronary that is as serious as other forms of heart attacks, but occurs without pain. That very same day, laboratory tests revealed that he was also diabetic.

I was not surprised at the doctor's findings, but I was dumbfounded by Dad's own prognosis. "Who told you that you have only four years?" I asked. He was silent for a long time, then said, "I just know."

His foreboding was true. He died four years later— almost to the day. It was a turning point in my life, the first of my two greatest losses. Sam Keen, author of *Your*

Mythic Journey and longtime friend of Joseph Campbell, is correct: until one's father dies, "there are giants in the world."

What happened during the four years that preceded my father's death was unexpected. At the time, I did not understand the extent to which a heart attack or a life-threatening illness can affect personality and invade all aspects of a person's life. Nor did I realize that the opposite is also true: that a heart attack or life-threatening illness can bring new and deeper meaning to life.

Seven years after my father's death I returned to graduate school. For eight years I juggled pursuing graduate studies, running a business, completing a dissertation, and being a husband and father. Eventually, I earned both an M.A. and Ph.D. in psychology.

During the last years of my graduate work I was fortunate to have Rachel Naomi Remen (a psychotherapist and cofounder of Commonweal, a retreat for persons with terminal illness) as my advisor and dissertation chair. There is an oriental saying, "When the student is ready, the teacher will come along." Naomi was the teacher who came into my life at precisely the right time. She nurtured and, at times, prodded gently. And without realizing it, I was back on track, trying to understand what happens to feelings of self-worth as we grow older and confront life-threatening illnesses.

My work with the elderly spans almost four decades:

First as a developer and manager of retirement communities; then, briefly after graduate school, as a psychotherapist; and finally as a part-time teacher at both Spring Hill College, where I was cofounder of the gerontology certificate program, and at the University of South Alabama.

This book emerged from a long-standing notion on my part that the experience of being an elder is more than can be comprehended by gerontology or, for that matter, by psychology or sociology. The social sciences are important in this endeavor, but they are not enough. What is required is a spiritual dimension, but not of the cloying and unctuous variety so often found in works on religion and aging. Hence my decision to rely heavily on the actual words of the elderly people who were my interviewees, and, as much as possible, to avoid academic or professional jargon.

In a nutshell this book deals with two questions: Which characteristics, environmental circumstances, or personal experiences cause the differences among elderly persons in feelings of self-worth, especially in the face of life-threatening illnesses? And why are some people deepened spiritually and psychologically by life-threatening illnesses, while others are disheartened and chronically demoralized?

Chapter One, "In the Land of the Young," is about the ambivalent feelings, seemingly common in America today, toward growing old. It contrasts the pessimistic view of great literature with the optimistic view that is prevalent in present-day gerontology.

The second chapter is about self-esteem, the linch-pin of how we feel about ourselves. Chapter Three is about *joss*, an oriental term that refers to a sense of pervasive good fortune; it concludes with a section on optimism and self-esteem.

Chapter Four is about the importance of what we say to ourselves. I chose the term *Doppelganger* rather than "self talk." A Doppelganger is the ghostly double that is always with us—the Me that I can never get rid of. (In an oddly similar way, it is the name that German sailors once gave to their duffel bags.)

Memories, and how they can nurture, heal, or lacerate the soul, are the subject of Chapter Five. Chapter Six is about trust, and about the wisdom of balancing personal independence with at least a modicum of healthy reliance upon others.

Chapter Seven is about perceptions of money and self-esteem. Chapter Eight is about partially disengaging, "letting go" of the activities of the past. Loneliness, and how it can kill, is the subject of Chapter Nine, which concludes with some reflections on the relationship between well-being and the sound of the human voice.

The influence of the male parent on self-esteem and, in turn, on perceptions of God as forgiving and loving, or punitive and vengeful, is the subject of Chapter Ten.

The next chapter is about the many masks that each of us wears, and the importance of one's "last call" for authenticity in the years of late life. The final chapter is about the wisdom of foolishness, and the importance of a touch of winsomeness to spiritual and psychological wholeness.

The chapters in this book are simply a way of organizing clues. People leave clues as they age. This is as true of life stories as it is of detective thrillers. The clues left by someone who is aging gently and graciously are different than those left by someone who feels the despair of a life lived with little in the way of self-esteem. To make it more complicated, although infinitely more interesting, even people who age gently seldom, if ever, do so in an absolute sense. "There is," as Emerson says, "a crack in everything God has made." Each reader must evaluate these clues according to his or her own circumstance. It is my hope that the clues will shed at least a little light on this, the most precious and mysterious of all blessings: the gift of a long life.

A Note to the Reader

Comments about, and references to, individual heart attack survivors demonstrating either high or low self-esteem are the result of a combination of in-depth interviews and two highly regarded self-esteem questionnaires. They are described in the appendix. Needless to say, anonymity has been ensured by changing the names of the interviewees, as well as references to geographic places.

Also, this book utilizes numerous quotations to illustrate various points. We have, in quotations throughout the book, taken the liberty of indicating emphasis by the use of *italics*.

Kind hearts are more than coronets,
And simple faith than Norman blood.

—Tennyson, English poet
laureate

A pure heart, remember, doesn't mean that you are a pure person. God save us from pure people. A pure heart is a good heart, an honest heart. It means that you have stopped hiding. It means you have stopped pretending to be pure, but have actually become pure by acknowledging your impurities.

—Albert Kreinheder, director
emeritus of the C. G. Jung
Institute of Los Angeles

Chapter 1

In the Land of the Young

> When asked why he had taken up the study of Greek at the age of eighty, the Roman statesman Cato the Elder replied, "It is the only age I have."

Our generation of elders is unlike other generations of elders. It is the first generation of full-timers. It is also the first generation of elders with true political clout.

Demographics alone have made America's older adults a population to be reckoned with, in terms of health care, housing, and quality of life. There are enough members in the American Association of Retired Persons (AARP) to form the thirtieth most populous country in the world, with almost as many people as Argentina.

Life expectancy in the United States has increased from 47 years in 1900 to more than 75 years in 1990.[1] At no other time in history has the news of someone dying at the age of 70 evoked a response about *dying young.* Old age is no longer a rarity. It is expected.

The meaning of old age has also changed. A 20-year-old may still think of 65 as old. But unless there is a disabling illness, a 65-year-old today is likely to be functioning at a level closer to midlife than to late adulthood. Thus the tendency of gerontology toward age subcategories: young-old (75 years or less), middle-old (76 to 84), and old-old (85 and older). Nonetheless, in spite of demographics, science, and popular writings that attest that old age isn't what it used to be, many timeworn notions remain. And timeworn notions have seldom been kind to the elderly.[2]

It isn't that the elderly, as individuals, are not loved and revered by family and friends. They are. Negative feelings are not about specific persons, but about old age itself. Robert C. Atchley, professor of social gerontology at Miami University, wrote:

> When we are dealing with specific older people in specific social roles, age is seldom seen as a negative trait. But when we deal with older people *as a social category*, especially in terms of social policy, we tend to do so in terms of negative images.[3]

Ambivalent images, rather than *negative* images, may be a description that is closer to the mark.

John, a 73-year-old friend of mine who is a lawyer by training, had an experience that typifies such ambivalence. John, whose career included representing a Fortune 500 company in Washington, D.C., for more than twenty years, and serving for several years as president of the Associated Industries of Alabama, had become bored with retirement. He needed a new quest.

At my suggestion, John and I met for lunch with the manager of our local business-development agency, a woman in her early thirties. John seemed to be the ideal person to promote new businesses. Many of his younger associates had become the decision-makers for their corporations. Several were personal friends. Since the manager seemed impressed, I had little doubt that some arrangement could be worked out, especially since John agreed to work for expenses only, with no salary.

The lunch meeting ended. As we stood up to say goodbye, the young woman, holding John's hand, said, "We would love to have you help us. Is Thursday good for you? Can you come in the morning? That's when the older men come to the office to help stuff envelopes and lick stamps."

During our long drive home, I broke the silence by telling John that the young woman only meant for him to come by Thursday morning to meet the other volunteers, and that she didn't expect someone with his credentials to "stuff envelopes and lick stamps." There was a long pause. Then John said, "Maybe. But I don't think so, and I'm sure as hell not going over there Thursday morning to find out."

Not being liked is not the problem; nor is being ignored. Nor are there many instances in which an older person is intentionally demeaned. It's simply not being welcomed, or even allowed, into the *circle*; and that in itself can nullify a sense of personhood, if one allows it. Such experiences underscore the importance of refusing to be treated as a second-class human being, even if it means occasional outbursts of orneriness or feistiness. It is an attitude aptly described by British elders as "bloody-mindedness."

The concept of the *circle* was well illustrated at a dinner party I know of. Prior to dinner, three couples were seated in the living room, talking, laughing, telling stories, and enjoying themselves. The chair arrangement formed an oval pattern, perfect for conversation. But not perfect for the hostess's mother—she sat in a chair behind her daughter, out of the circle.

Anthropologists Margaret Clark and Barbara Anderson wrote more than twenty-five years ago, in *Culture and Aging: An Anthropological Study of Older Americans*, that people must learn to identify at what point in time their culture expects them to grow old, and how to do it. Otherwise their last years will be fraught with difficulties.[4]

Ambivalent or negative images of the elderly are usually tacit and insidious, as is sometimes seen in discussions about health-care reform. Thorny issues such as rationed health care—determining, literally, who lives and who dies—are often leveled in the direction of the very old. Consider, as an example, an announcement in 1999 that the state of Oregon would subsidize assisted suicide for individuals who are indigent.[5] The stress that such an option could place on patient, family, and physician is unimaginable.

Ambivalent feelings toward the old, and, frequently, the old toward one another, are made somewhat clearer by comparing the dire perceptions of old age that are found in religion, great literature, and theater on the one hand, with the more optimistic findings of social gerontology on the other.

References in the Bible to old age, for example, are more enigmatic than double-edged. There is, of course, the voyeuristic story of Susanna and the two elders in the Book of Daniel.[6]

In that story (found only in Catholic versions of the Bible), two self-righteous elders lust after Susanna. They find her alone at her bath and threaten to turn her over to the authorities for the crime of adultery unless she yields to their desires. She refuses. The two elders give false testimony and Susanna is condemned to death. Daniel, at the time a young man, is moved by the Holy Spirit to stop the execution. He cross-examines the two elders and traps them in their lie. Susanna's life is spared and she returns to her husband. The two elders, however, do not fare as well. Under the Law of Moses, both are sentenced to death.

Other than that story, however, there are no incidents that associate old age with vice rather than virtue. The Hebrew Scriptures could not have been clearer: "Honor your father and your mother as Yahweh your God has commanded you, so that you may have long life and may prosper in the land that Yahweh your God gives to you."[7]

Still, the ordeal of being old, and the frustrations that come with caring for the elderly, resonate through the centuries, as the Psalmist cries out, "Cast me not off in the time of old age; forsake me not when my strength faileth."[8] More wrenching, and perhaps reflective of the attitude of the time, is the admonition to the young that is found in Ecclesiastes, "And remember your Creator in the days of your youth, before evil days come and the years approach when you say, 'These give me no pleasure. . . .'" The authors of that work regarded the buffeting that the old endured as one of humankind's greatest misfortunes. Stark and abject horror are felt as Ecclesiastes continues, ". . . when the sound of the mill is faint, when the voice of the bird is silenced, and the song notes are stilled, when to go uphill is an ordeal and a walk is something to dread."[9]

In Roman times, the dread of old age was ritualized. Wall paintings that survived the destruction of Pompeii in 79 A.D. depict an initiation in which a young man looks into a mirror. Instead of his own handsome face, he sees the face of an old man. "This is you," the elder initiators told him. And, because of the power of the ritual, the young man, perhaps for the first time, confronted the inevitability of old age.

Today there are no rituals. There are retirement-planning seminars, but such seminars are oriented to the head rather than the heart. The need for ritual, however, persists. Teachers of gerontology often hear of this need, articulated in the answers of students who, when asked why they are taking the course, reply that they are preparing for their own old age.

The theater, frequently the medium of the otherwise unspeakable, deals more directly with feelings toward the old. For the most part, the elderly are objects of derision, as in *Aristophanes and Plautus*, where the character of the old man is presented as a dehumanized "other," a source of laughter and derision. The old man is not a person but an object, a projection of our dread of old age.

Centuries later, the commedia dell'arte, a form of Italian comedy, had, as a common motif, an old man cuckolded by his pretty young wife—a just and moral comeuppance, so to speak. Sexuality in which an old man and a young woman are lovers is still seen as both disdainful and disgusting; that is, unless you happen to be the old man in question!

A friend of mine who was in his 60s was asked by a female colleague in her late 20s if he would have an affair with a 25-year-old woman, if given the chance.

When he answered yes, she expressed shock and dismay, and gasped, "I can't believe my ears."

Indicative of the depths from which such allegedly unfitting behaviors emerge is the absence of a slang equivalent of the phrase "dirty old man" for an elderly woman who lusts after young men. A "dirty old woman" is too repugnant for words, even in our day. I do not remember ever hearing anyone use that phrase, even to describe the lustiest of old women.

In Elizabethan theater, truths that were expressed by the elderly, no matter how profound, were regarded as tiresome, as in Hamlet's pejorative toward Polonious: "These tedious old fools!" Or, later in the play, Rosencrantz's comment, to this day the bane of enlightened gerontology: ". . . they say an old man is twice a child."[10] If the old dare do what is considered unfitting, as in Falstaff's sexual escapades, they are ridiculed.

On the other hand, there are few instances in which we so poignantly come face to face with our last and ultimate selves as in *King Lear*:

> O' Sir, you are old;
> Nature in you stands on the very verge
> Of her confine. You should be ruled and led
> By some discretion that discerns your state
> Better than you yourself.[11]

In the play, daughter Regan takes her father's power

and all that goes with it, leaving Lear the trappings of an empty kingship. Shakespeare's tragedy brings to mind our elders, who are, in an oddly similar manner, divested of their place in society by family or by court-mandated conservatorships. Or the experiences of people who are not quite ready to retire, but are laid off because of a corporate downsizing.

Old age, according to geriatrician M. Grotjahn, is more of a cultural artifact than a biological reality. To the younger generation, especially in America, our elders are "the representatives of the dark past."[12] This is not a new idea. The same observation was made by Jonathan Swift more than 250 years ago. In *Gulliver's Travels*, Swift described the Struldbruggs, people who lived to extreme old age, as having "the disadvantage of living like foreigners in their own country."[13]

Negative feelings that come with age are felt more deeply by women than men. Elissa Melamed, a psychotherapist, likened the afternoon of a woman's life to the dark side of the moon:

> It is the side facing away from the world, man's world, and is therefore the half that is unknown, invisible, and often ignored. It can be the dark and difficult side of life for many women on whom the sun shined in their youth.[14]

In the late 1970s, *Playboy* magazine featured an

article about the mystique of the older woman. All but one of the women who were featured were in their early to mid-30s. The single exception was a woman about to turn 40. Women older than 40 were apparently not considered sexy.

At this point the argument about ambivalence toward, and negative stereotyping of, the elderly takes a strange turn. In spite of great literature, scripture, the theater, etc., the prevailing opinion of social gerontology is that most of our elders are reasonably pleased with the quality of their lives.

The pithy comment of nineteenth-century French author and diplomat Chateaubriand, "Old age is a shipwreck,"[15] simply doesn't ring true. Or, more accurately, it doesn't ring true unless or until—and this is the key issue—a person experiences an illness that is chronic and disabling to the point of significantly impairing actual, or perceived, quality of life. Even then, the impact of chronic and disabling illness upon quality of life is often less devastating than imagined.

In 1987 the U.S. Senate Special Committee on Aging reported that more than four out of five community-dwelling elders (that is, elders not living in nursing homes or other institutions) had at least one chronic illness. Nonetheless, of those with chronic illnesses, only one in four described his or her condition as disabling to a significant degree. And of the one in four, fewer than two percent were bedridden.[16]

The bottom line is that most of our elders, including those with chronic illnesses, manage to get along nicely. They may not drive at night; they may be slow in performing certain tasks such as cooking, housekeeping, shopping, etc. But they are not inconvenienced in a major way, nor are they displeased with their lives. Barring significant functional impairment, such as being housebound or unable to fend for one's self in even minimal ways, there is much in late life to look forward to.

Most of the adages about being over 65 are simply not true; for example, people do not die as a result of retiring. To the contrary, the majority of retirees describe their health as good. Many feel that they are in better health than before they retired. The occasional retiree that dies shortly after retirement usually dies of the illness that prompted the decision to retire. Nor do marriages deteriorate because both spouses are home together all day long. Some marriages actually get better.[17]

The viewpoints of religion, theater, great literature, etc., and social gerontology seem to be 180 degrees opposite. Gerontology gives new meaning to an old story from the Muslim mystic tradition called Sufism:

> Two lawyers are arguing a case. After the first

lawyer's summary, the judge says, "You're right." After the second lawyer's summary, the judge again says, "You're right." The two lawyers leap to their feet and shout in unison, "Both of us can't be right." The judge replies, "You're right."[18]

The difference is in the *truths* of religion, great literature, and theater versus the *truths* of social gerontology. The latter typically relies on empirical research—findings that can be quantified and supported statistically. The truths of the former are quite different: they do not lend themselves to statistical validation. They are where the heart is.

It is not that one position is correct and the other isn't. Both are correct. It is, rather, that as we grow older we look at the inequities of life in a new light. Judith Viorst, a best-selling author trained in psychology, wrote:

> There also may be a shift in the way we perceive the hard times in our life—a shift from "tragedy" to "irony." Tragedy is all-encompassing and all black. . . . Irony sees the same event written a little smaller. Its blackness doesn't fill the entire screen. This shift in perception from tragedy to irony may be the special gift of our late years, helping us to deal with our accumulating losses, and sometimes also helping us to grow.[19]

The shift from tragedy to irony has a numinous, mys-

Kind Hearts

terious quality. It evokes what American psychologist Rollo May called the *wonderful* in human beings, as in the attitudes of two people I interviewed several years ago. Each had had a heart attack and, later, coronary artery bypass surgery.

The first is a 72-year-old man whose wife is confined to bed because of osteoporosis and scoliosis; the second is a 76-year-old widow who is the sole support of an alcohol-dependent middle-aged son. Each is worried about what will become of the dependent loved one who, more than likely, will outlive them. Nonetheless, they not only maintain a positive outlook but, for reasons individual to each, regard their illnesses as having enriched their lives. Both described an enhanced awareness of how precious life is, and the importance of living it fully. One said that her heart attack saved her life, by freeing her from commitments that placed the well-being of others above her own needs.[20]

The distinguished Swiss psychiatrist Carl G. Jung, writing of his own heart attack, which occurred at the age of 69, had much the same response:

> Something else, too, came from my illness. I might formulate it as an affirmation of things as they are: an unconditional "yes" to that which is, without subjective protests— acceptance of the conditions of existence as I see them and understand them; acceptance of my own nature, as I happen to be.[21]

The Irish poet W. B. Yeats, in "The Coming of Wisdom with Time," said, gently and delicately, much the same about his old age:

> Though leaves are many, the root is one;
> Through all the lying days of my youth
> I swayed my leaves and flowers in the sun;
> Now I may wither into the truth.[22]

Chapter 2

What We Feel About Ourselves (Self-Esteem)

"My mother once said to me, 'If you decide to become a soldier you will be a general, if you decide to become a priest you will become a Pope . . .' Well, instead, I decided to become an artist and I became Picasso."

> —Pablo Picasso, painter and sculptor

Humility is the proper pursuit of one's own excellence.

> —St. Thomas Aquinas, 13th-century Catholic theologian

Self-esteem is a household word. It is a mainstay of popular psychology. Fortunately its meaning has survived the transition from the academic world to the everyday world relatively intact. In either world, high self-esteem implies respect for oneself and a sense of worthiness. In contrast, low self-esteem implies self-rejection and feelings of unworthiness.[1]

The presence or absence of self-esteem permeates almost every aspect of life. Self-esteem is regarded by some psychologists as the "most powerful and pervasive role in higher life"[2] and "co-extensive with life itself."[3] Ernest Becker, the existential writer and teacher, went a step further in linking it to heroism: "Everything painful and sobering, in what psychoanalytic genius and religious genius discovered about man, revolves around the terror of admitting what one is doing to earn his self-esteem."[4]

Although self-esteem in the elderly is much like self-esteem at other ages, there are important differences. Most of the differences are external and reflect cultural and social views of aging: youth, vigor, wealth, and wrinkle-free skin are too frequently identified as indices of how we should feel about ourselves.

Self-esteem in the elderly often evokes images of super-achievers: a select group of people, the people whose photos appear in high-style magazines. The pervasiveness of this attitude even extends to those working in the social sciences. A psychologist, when told of my interest in self-esteem in the elderly, asked, half seriously, "Does one of them actually have it?"

An experiment illustrated some of the difficulties that the elderly face in maintaining self-esteem. Photographs of the same man at ages 25, 52, and 73 were shown to a sampling of traditional-age college students.[5] The students rated the man at each of the three

Kind Hearts

ages for nineteen characteristics, ranging from intelligence and creativity to competence and social involvement. The photo of the man at 73 was rated *significantly* lower (as defined statistically) in all of the characteristics except generosity. He was also lowest in generosity, but not significantly so.

Still, gerontologists affirm that, except under the most trying of circumstances, self-esteem is not lowered by either aging per se or by the onset of most age-related illnesses. Nor do age and illness serve as barometers of individual circumstances. John Rowe, who heads the MacArthur Foundation, aptly commented, "I can describe to you a 75-year-old man with a history of heart disease and diabetes, and you can't tell me with any confidence whether he will be sitting on the Supreme Court or in a nursing home."[6]

Self-esteem is often confused with self-concept. Although closely related, the two are separate and distinct. Self-concept, as the term implies, relates to concepts, ideas, and facts. It doesn't matter whether they are right or wrong, true or false. They are still the concepts, ideas, and facts that we believe about ourselves. I think of myself as a husband, father, business person, teacher, animal lover, member of the Jung Society, and responsible for a house mortgage. I am competent, regarded favorably by most of my students, and loved by my wife, three children, a dog, and four cats. This is my self-concept, sketchy but descriptive. However, it does not tell me how I *feel* about myself.

Self-esteem, on the other hand, does not describe. Self-esteem is a visceral, deep down, gut-level feeling. It tells me how I *feel* about myself. The fact that I feel good about myself may be incomprehensible in the eyes of others. It may fly in the face of common sense, but that doesn't matter. It is a feeling, not a concept or fact. I may be an indifferent father, an insensitive husband, a teacher who grades subjectively, an individual with few redeeming qualities, and still have high self-esteem. By the same token, the reverse may be true. I may be all that my culture and upbringing says that I should be, but still have low self-esteem.[7]

Each "self" term can influence the other and go awry, as in a story told about John Steinbeck. After reading the galley proofs of his masterpiece, *The Grapes of Wrath*, Steinbeck became profoundly depressed. He not only *felt* that the book was mediocre, but that after years of hard work, mediocrity *was the best he was capable of.*

A less serious example, involving people's skewed perceptions of self, occurred in a large southwestern city. A film company announced a call for "beautiful people" and asked that they assemble in a downtown plaza on a Saturday morning. Hundreds of people showed up. Photos of them were taken and submitted to a panel of judges. Of the hundreds of people, the judges found that only a few were even remotely good-

Kind Hearts

looking, to say nothing of being either beautiful or handsome. The vast majority were quite ordinary. Some were rated as grossly unattractive, even ugly. But, apparently, they all *felt* beautiful.

Deepak Chopra wrote, "Our way of looking at ourselves makes us what we are. If we could change our way of looking, we could in fact change all notions, and therefore all realities, of living, aging, mortality, and ultimately immortality—*for it is our notions that construct those realities.*"8

Almost two thousand years ago the Greek stoic philosopher Epictetus said much the same thing: "Man is not disturbed by things, but by his opinion of things."9 William James, still regarded by many as one of America's premier psychologists, emphasized the importance of our *notions* to the value we place on specific abilities or aspects of our lives:

> I, who for the time have staked my all on being a psychologist, am mortified if others know more about psychology than I. But I am contented to wallow in the grossest ignorance of Greek. My deficiencies there give me no sense of personal humiliation at all. Had I "pretensions" to be a linguist, it would have been just the reverse.10

One characteristic of high or low self-esteem is the way in which we compare ourselves to people our same age, and/or to people in similar circumstances. The comparisons may be more than casual or superficial—they may affect health, wellness, and even life itself. In a study of women with breast cancer, psychologist Shelly Taylor found that a favorable comparison to another woman with breast cancer was one of the three predictors of successful recovery.[11]

Other comparisons are less straightforward. Some are perplexing, even humorous, and on the surface make no sense at all. At a deeper level, however, such comparisons may serve as protectors from, or buffers against, the negative stereotypes associated with old age. Examples of comparisons heard among residents of retirement communities include:

> I'm not like those other women. I don't blame men for not looking at them.

> [Reaction to a confused resident.] He shouldn't be allowed to live here. It depresses the rest of us who have our marbles.

> [Comment of a resident with a severe tremor caused by Parkinson's disease, about another resident who uses a walker.] They ought to kick her out of the dining room. She belongs in the nursing home. She depresses the rest of us. Thank God, I've got my health.

> [An 82-year-old real estate executive during a visit to a retirement community.] Will you look at those old bastards in the dining room! I guess somebody has to take care of them!

At times we are not aware of comparisons. I was having a more difficult time than others in my ta'i chi ch'uan (Tai Chi) class. The gentle, dancelike exercises were more formidable than I had anticipated, but I didn't think I was doing too badly. Then my ineptness was brought home to me. A woman, who was a contemporary of mine, told me that, since I had joined the class, everyone else felt much better about how they were doing.

People with high self-esteem seem to place more value on mental attributes and learned skills than on physical attractiveness and athletic ability.[12] Richard, a man in his mid-70s, told of always being challenged by new interests:

> Life is not boring to me. I don't mean there aren't hours when I don't have something to do, but life is never boring. My wife says I go to the library and she never knows what kind of books I'm going to bring home. I'm continually getting new interests. Like our trip to Muir Woods . . . I got interested in ecology, forestry, and geology. Something continually ignites new interests.

Responses of interviewees with low self-esteem were quite different. The most moving response was from a woman who had won dozens of trophies as a ballroom dancer. There was sadness in her eyes as she leafed through albums of photographs taken when she was in her 30s and 40s. One photograph showed her crying. She said she was crying because she had not yet learned to do the tango, and "everyone else was dancing."

A retired insurance executive with low self-esteem said he valued his athletic abilities more than anything else. He was an amateur baseball player until his late 40s:

> Baseball, basketball, and football. I was better than average. But when I got sick I didn't think I could do anything again . . . which I couldn't. I was so doggone weak I couldn't hardly move. I can't even make up my mind to get out there and cut the yard yet . . . and I used to have this place looking like an estate . . . when I was in the garden, before, I was king.

This man's unhappiness was reinforced by his physician. When asked for "permission" (his word) to go fishing, the physician told him that it was okay, provided he cranked the motor of his outboard only once. "If it doesn't start the first time, get in your car and drive home. It's too risky to crank it twice."

A retired business owner, recently divorced from his wife of more than forty years, was critical of "overeducated college professors with no common sense."

Another, a delightful man, valued his attractiveness to women more than anything else. At the beginning of the interview I asked if there was anything that, on a daily basis, reminded him of his heart attack. He tapped the center of his chest with his finger and said, "Not really. There's a little pain here. But it has nothing to do with the heart. They call it vagina! . . . Damn, I meant angina!" But later in the interview he told me that his life "went to hell for good" in his early 50s when he became impotent. He sought medical help, but his physician told him that he couldn't expect anything else at his age. He was silent for a moment before saying that his wife "teases" him about it. (Spare us from such physicians and spouses!)

Moral competence, too, is entwined with self-esteem. Not, however, in the sense of high or low moral values. Most of the people I interviewed prided themselves on their integrity. Each could recall good feelings that came from not taking the easy way. The difference was that persons with low self-esteem seemed to equate moral competence with personal sacrifice and self-denial. Their responses recalled the comments of author and psychotherapist Dennis Jaffe about the self-defeating behavior of people who sacrifice their most basic needs to the well-being of others:

> So many of my patients have experienced a neglect of their most basic, deepest human needs—for touching and for companionship, for sharing inner feelings, for expressing creative energy, for sexual fulfillment, for per-

sonal validation, and for giving and receiving love. Instead, their lives were characterized by duty and obligation to the very people who gave them nothing in return.[13]

The heart attack survivors with high self-esteem did not lose sight of their personal needs. They took better care of themselves, physically and emotionally. Robert, whose wife of fifty years suffers from schizophrenia, comes to mind. He did not want to dissolve the marriage. Nor did he want to give up the happiness and pleasure he received from other aspects of his life. "I had to put the problems with my wife out of my mind . . . otherwise I'd be miserable. I can't do anything about it . . . [a long pause] I made it a practice not to worry about things I can't do anything about."

Robert described his heart attack as "a blessing in disguise" that not only resulted in a commitment to physical health, but got him "to thinking about God." As Naomi Remen observed, a life-threatening illness turns us into seekers.[14]

Optimism and humor were guardians of Robert's sense of self-worth as he described his recovery at home following coronary artery bypass surgery: "You don't know how fast you can get better and go back to work until you're married to a woman who keeps talking about a tunnel the communists are digging under the house."

Without question, aging, especially after ages 65 or

70, impinges upon most aspects of life. There are losses. But there are also compensations, sometimes even gains, both psychologically and spiritually. Borrowing James's global concept of *self*, and applying it to what happens in late adulthood, helps bring the losses, compensations, and gains into sharper focus.

James defined the self as the sum of all that each of us can call his or her own. The self, he said, has three constituent parts: the *material Me*, the *social Me*, and the *spiritual Me*.[15]

The Material Me

The material Me refers to one's body, family, and possessions—material entities that, by sentiment or ownership, give a sense of personal wholeness. The elderly face an erosion of the material Me with declining health, loss of spouse, deaths of friends, reduction of income, or moving from a cherished home.

Fortunately, the significance of an eroding material Me is much different in late adulthood than earlier in life. This is especially so in the responses of the elderly to questions about living on a reduced income. Contrary to the expectations of younger adults, most retirees are satisfied with their retirement incomes, even though their incomes may be significantly less than their earnings before retirement. Gerontologists attribute this to a combination of things, including a self-preserving tendency of our elders to modify their views of what constitutes an adequate income.

In other words, retirees tend to reframe their earlier aspirations in order to conform more closely to the realities of their individual circumstances.[16] As James wrote more than a century ago, ". . . to give up pretensions is as blessed a relief as to get them gratified; and where disappointment is incessant and the struggle unending, this is what men will always do."[17]

The attenuation of the material Me affects each of us differently. It is harsh and heart-rending to some of our elders, especially those who are forced to move to nursing homes. However, among others, especially more-affluent retirees, the attenuation of the material Me is generally pleasant. A cherished home, for example, may be replaced by a smaller home or condominium, often located in a Sun Belt area with beaches and golf courses nearby.

The material Me of more-affluent retirees has not gone unnoticed. Marketing to seniors has become a Madison Avenue specialty. Its proponents boast that no age group equals America's elderly in spendable income. But there are occasional surprises, as in a video that promoted sponsorship for a TV series geared to seniors living in Florida. A saccharine description of America's elderly was shattered when one of the marketing experts said, "I tell you, about ten years ago if you asked someone what a senior citizen is like, we'd look at an old lady or old man eating dog or cat food."[18] (Who can doubt that Madison Avenue has at last stumbled upon salvation!)

The Social Me

The social Me is located in the minds of others. There is not a single social Me, but as many social Me's as there are persons who carry an image of the individual in their minds. James's social Me anticipated what Charles H. Cooley, a sociologist who lived early in the twentieth century, described as the "looking glass self."[19] The "looking glass self" places self-esteem in our beliefs about how we are perceived by others.

The social Me is diminished simply by outliving friends and acquaintances. I interviewed a man in his late 70s who not only named his deceased friends, as if at roll call, but also the causes of their deaths and the names of their physicians!

The social Me of residents who move to full-service retirement communities fares better. These individuals live longer and get sick less frequently.[20] One reason may be the presence and companionship of other people, a replenishment of the social Me.

The Spiritual Me

James's third constituent part, the spiritual Me, refers to one's inner or subjective being. It incorporates not only the present, the "here and now," but the experiences and feelings of a lifetime. It resembles what Erik Erikson,[21] a psychoanalyst and life-stage development theorist, regarded as the ultimate task of late life: the integration of the properties of the ego (or conscious mind). Thus, the term chosen by Erikson—*ego integrity*.

Ego integrity is a bone-deep feeling that the sum of one's life—all that has happened, good and bad—somehow makes sense, and that one's life could not have been lived in any other way. Further, that one's life, just as it was lived, made a difference, however small, in the universal order of things.

If ego integrity is lacking, its absence will be felt by a sense of despair, an arching and horrible realization in one's last years that life should have been lived differently, but now it is too late. Despair is the feeling of having been on the wrong quest or, perhaps worse, on no quest at all. It is the angst of Charley's eulogy at Willy Loman's funeral in Arthur Miller's play *Death of a Salesman*:

> He's a man way out there in the blue, riding on a smile and a shoeshine. And when they start not smiling back—that's an earthquake. And then you get yourself a couple of spots on your hat and you're finished.[22]

Few persons complete the task of ego integration in its fullest sense: Gandhi, Eleanor Roosevelt, and Thomas

Merton (the Trappist monk and author) are world-recognized individuals that come to mind. Most of us, however, do quite well if the balance is weighted in the direction of ego integrity rather than despair. C. G. Jung wrote:

> But we must not forget that only a very few people are artists in life; that the art of life is the most distinguished and rarest of all the arts. Who ever succeeded in draining the whole cup with grace?[23]

The question is, Can feelings of self-worth be raised from low to high? I think the answer is yes. Even in late life it is possible to raise feelings of self-worth and set aside feelings of unworthiness, but it is hard work. Most people resist change with their whole heart. The poet W. H. Auden wrote:

> We would rather be ruined than changed;
> We would rather die in our dread
> Than climb the cross of the moment
> And let our illusions die.[24]

Sheldon Kopp, author of that enduring classic on the pilgrimage of psychotherapy, *If You Meet the Buddha on the Road, Kill Him!*, said that, time and again, patients insist that they want to change, but in fact want only to be made more-effective neurotics. They prefer "the security of known misery to the misery of unfamiliar insecurity."[25]

The following chapters flesh out the importance of self-esteem as it affects, and is in turn affected by, opinions and beliefs, ranging from trust and money to parental relationships and perceptions of God.

To feel good about oneself after a lifetime of feeling unworthy is a great achievement at any age, a very heroic act in anyone's book. But for those who are willing to suffer and endure the hard work of self-knowledge, the rewards are great. Not the least of the rewards is an unblocking of psychic energy that, in turn, frees one to accept what Joseph Campbell, the twentieth century's most celebrated authority on comparative mythology, called the gifts of *invisible hands*, gifts akin to *joss* or feelings of pervasive good fortune, and the subject of the next chapter.

Chapter 3

Joss, the I'Ching, and Explanatory Style

Until he is dead, do not call a man happy, but only lucky.

> —Herodotus, ancient Greek historian

Tell the boys I've got the luck with me now.

> —Brett Harte, American writer

Good fortune is a god among men, and more than god.

> —Aeschylus, ancient Greek dramatist

Joss is a Chinese word that means good luck or good fortune of a special kind; good luck or good fortune that is *pervasive* and *omnipresent*. A person with joss simply runs in good luck. If you have it, there is an angel on your shoulder. Without question you are blessed.

Joss is defined by the American Heritage Dictionary as a Chinese idol. Its derivation is Pidgin English, from the Portuguese for *Deus* or *God*. A *joss house* is a small temple with an idol. In Weaverville, California, there is a joss house built by the Chinese immigrants who worked in nearby mines more than a century ago. It can be visited to this day.

For those of us rooted in a Western way of looking at things, the full significance of joss may be elusive. A life that is guided, protected, and sometimes manipulated by external forces is, at first blush, incomprehensible. The possibility of a life that is influenced by events that are acausal, but nonetheless ordered, simply does not fit into our world. It may even seem unfair.

By the same token, we sometimes speak of someone whose life has been *blessed*, or someone who has experienced the presence of *grace*. Grace is familiar to us; it is a part of Christian theology and is acknowledged by people of all denominations. It is the subject of the beloved hymn "Amazing Grace." Grace and joss are similar. Grace is rooted in the Christian tradition; joss in the Oriental tradition.

To a greater or lesser degree, each of us has wondered about powers that we do not understand. Even the detractors of events or facts that cannot be rationally explained tread lightly when it comes to luck or destiny. "God is on the side with the heaviest artillery," said Napoleon Bonaparte, acknowledging the zeitgeist of the day. Still, the question he asked of each young officer who wanted to be his adjutant was, "Is he lucky?"

Now to get to the point. In listening to the taped interviews of elderly heart attack survivors, certain words and phrases were repeated time and again. However, the words and phrases were different among high self-esteem versus low self-esteem interviewees. High self-esteem interviewees, without exception, at some point in the interview, referred to themselves as lucky or fortunate or blessed; and, most important, lucky or fortunate or blessed in a pervasive sense.[1] Thus the analogy to joss.

In describing his heart attack, Allen, a 74-year-old man, said:

> We came back from fishing, had a drink or two, and lunch. After lunch the pains got worse, so they [friends] put me in bed and I began to perspire and he [a friend] called the ambulance. I was so very *fortunate*, the ambulance was already at [the town] and didn't have to come all the way from [nearby town with ambulance service]. I've always been lucky that way.

William, another interviewee, age 80, reminisced about when he worked for a major television network and had responsibility for the news coverage at national events. After talking about the pain of rheumatoid arthritis and saying that he no longer had the physical stamina for such work, he said:

> But I'm *lucky*. A bunch of us old TV and radio

guys get on the ham radio at four o'clock in the afternoon, five days a week. We talk about the old times, swap stories . . . sometimes help one another out. I get on two or three times a week and it's like us old cronies meeting in a beer joint.

George, a man in his mid-70s, is realistic about his illness. He too recognizes the limitations it has imposed upon him. Still, optimism and a sense of pervasive good fortune are obvious:

I've always had an optimistic outlook on life. I'm *fortunate* in that respect. I always felt the things you can't change, you have to accept and try to make the best of them. It's a handicap, I guess [points to his heart]. But more of an inconvenience than a handicap. I'm always able to do anything I want, within reason and moderation.

To an Oriental, joss is second nature. Acausal events are regarded as having their own incomprehensible cosmic order. They neither challenge nor detract from the rationale of cause and effect. The two simply coexist side by side. This is due in no small measure to a world view that is influenced by a 2,500-year-old book of divination called the *Book of Changes* or the *I'Ching*.

The *I'Ching* dates back to the Shang Dynasty, almost two thousand years before the birth of Jesus Christ. It evolved slowly. Much of its refinement was the work of

Confucius (551–479 B.C.), who devoted the last years of his life to studying and perfecting it.

The *I'Ching* consists of sixty-four hexagrams. Each hexagram represents a text that is identified by manipulating yarrow stalks or, alternatively, tossing three coins six times. Although the yarrow stalks are more cumbersome, they add a tactile dimension, reminding the seeker that the *I'Ching* reaches upward, just as the yarrow plant grows out of the earth toward the heavens. Each hexagram is a response to the seeker's question. Most baffling, of course, is the uncanny accuracy of a hexagram chosen by chance.

An anecdote: I was preparing a syllabus for my first graduate class in Jungian Psychology and Christianity at Spring Hill College. I had mixed feelings about including a section on the *I'Ching*. Spring Hill is a Jesuit college; the course was part of the Theology curriculum and, at the time, I was new to teaching. Most of all I did not want to be summarily fired. As the date for the lecture approached I became more and more apprehensive. Finally I decided to consult the *I'Ching* itself. I tossed the three coins six times and arrived at the hexagram named "Li." Included in its text was my answer:

> The great man continues the work of nature in the human world. Through the clarity of his nature he causes the light to spread farther and farther and to penetrate the nature of man ever more deeply.[2]

That was good enough for me. The students were fascinated and responded well. To this day, however, one of them still chides me because I refused to toss the coins or manipulate the yarrow stalks as part of a classroom demonstration.

The *I'Ching* is not a parlor game to be toyed with. No one understands how it works. It simply does. C. G. Jung wrote; "The less one thinks about the theory of the *I'Ching*, the more soundly one sleeps."[3]

At the heart of the *I'Ching* is a process spawned out of the Oriental psyche—*the chain of causation*. The rationale of the chain of causation is quite different than that of our Western concept of cause and effect. The latter is what it purports to be: one identifiable event causes another identifiable event to happen, and is therefore amenable to empirical testing. The chain of causation, on the other hand, relates to an interdependence among and between all things: a divine, omniscient, and harmonious linking of all that makes up the cosmos. It resonates to a phrase from the Nicene Creed, describing the vastness of God's creation as encompassing "all things, *seen* and *unseen*."

The chance selection of a hexagram that specifically applies to the seeker's question is a phenomenon that is related to *synchronicity*, a term that Jung used to describe acausal events or experiences. Synchronistic events are experiences that are connected through their meaning, but cannot be explained by cause and effect.

Kind Hearts

They are experiences that, based on laws of probability or chance, never should have happened. Synchronicity, to paraphrase psychiatrist Jean Shinoda Bolin, is what we call the link or connection between two or more experiences or events, when we can't call it anything else.[4]

Synchronistic events occur in many ways *if* (and this is all-important) we allow ourselves to be open to them. They are not planned. They simply happen. I, for example, frequently experience them on airplane trips. The reason, I think, is that I am at heart a "white knuckle" flyer, and abandon all pretense of what I imagine myself to be until the airplane is once again safely on the ground. (It takes less than five minutes of heavy turbulence to dissolve my ego-ideal and reduce my equanimity to rubble.)

My airplane synchronicity stories are many, and they always involve random seating assignments: for example, sitting next to a woman who was worried because she had to write five radio programs on aging, about which she knew nothing (I drafted an outline for her); listening to a woman's story about her father's sexual abuse of her daughter—a story, she said, that had to be told, but not to someone in the small town in which she lived (I was the perfect listener: trained in psychotherapy, anonymous, and never to be seen again). In each example the plane was crowded, and my preference for being surrounded by vacant seats gave way to being seated next to someone else.

Viewed over a lifetime, synchronistic events are similar to *pointillism*, a style of painting developed by the nineteenth-century French Impressionist George Seurat. A Seurat painting, seen from across the room, reflects a clear and easily recognized composition. But seen from one or two feet away, the composition clearly reveals itself as a mass of dots or points. To recognize synchronistic events, or, more important, to attract them, requires an openness or receptivity to their possibility: a stepping back, so to speak, as in viewing a Seurat painting. The same can be said of joss. Joss, too, requires openness and receptivity to the more positive qualities of life.

Greek myths are rich with synchronicity. They reveal a psychology that is as profound today as the day the myths were first told. The Greek god most often associated with synchronicity and acausal events is Hermes. Hermes plays many roles: the messenger of the gods, the guide for the dead in their journey to Hades, and, most important, the god who, in disguise, is sent to warn, redirect, or inspire the hero in his or her quest. Time and again, Hermes warned Odysseus of impending dangers during his travels. Hermes shielded King Priam as he wended his way through the Greek encampment, in the last days of the Trojan War, to plead for the body of his son, Hector, the mighty warrior slain by Achilles. Hermes is a mythic and dynamic expression of synchronicity. Interventions by Hermes mirrored joss.

The importance of having luck on your side extended even to Zeus, the most powerful god in the Greek pantheon. Zeus took no chances when it came to luck. Tyche, the goddess of luck, traveled everywhere at his side. "She is pictured on a constantly revolving wheel, and in her journeys around the world she 'scattered with careless hands her numerous gifts, lavishing with indifference her choicest smiles.'"[5] The Roman equivalent of Tyche is Fortune, whose symbol, a revolving wheel, resembles a roulette table.

Although each of the high self-esteem heart attack survivors made at least one reference to good fortune, good luck, or feeling blessed, those with low self-esteem were a different story. They used words such as cheated, betrayed, or stolen. A 74-year-old woman described the prospects of spending the remaining years of her life with her husband, a recovering alcoholic:

> We worked hard for this house and furniture. He's been cured and feels young. I'm afraid I'm going to die and he's going to find somebody to move in with him and I'll be *cheated* out of all we struggled for. Some other woman will get the house, the furniture, the boat . . . everything.

A respected local business owner retired from his

flourishing corporation and sold the business to his son. On the surface it seemed like the American dream. But he said that, apart from his business, life gave him little else. His marriage was empty and void of feeling—merely a contract of endurance. He described his wife's affection as an "occasional peck on the cheek if I was leaving on a business trip, nothing more." In spite of business success and memberships in prestigious country clubs, he regretted not staying in New York and pursuing his dream of working in the theater: "I would have loved any part of it . . . acting, directing, writing . . . I would have been happy building sets . . . even selling tickets."

He visits the office once a week but feels unhappy during the time he is there: "I write a letter or two, pay personal bills, and let the company pay for the postage." He wanted to retire years earlier but his senior vice president went to work for someone else: "We lost a man to [another company]. They *stole* him away by offering him a vice presidency and more money than I could pay him. I depended on him for so much. I had to keep working."

Interviewees with low self-esteem tended to perceive their world as hostile. "Reverse joss" seemed to follow them, hovering above like a dark cloud and eerily indifferent to material success, as in an interview that took place in an expensive home in the Buckhead area of Atlanta. The interviewee, a man in his mid-70s, told of working side by side with his wife to build up a business that ultimately sold for more than $2 million—a Horatio Alger story. Then his wife moved to Hawaii, filed for divorce, and *"got away with* an awful lot of liquid [assets] . . . that left the other partner with assets but no liquid." Later in the interview he said he was an easy mark:

> I used to be a softie, an easy touch . . . but I am about to grow out of that now . . . harden up a little bit . . . so many people nowadays will *take advantage of you* . . . People see what my wife *did to me* [the divorce settlement] and that it didn't seem to hurt me too bad . . . so they want a piece of the pie. Of course, I don't blame them.

Poignantly, after describing commitments to social and civic organizations, he related how busy he was having a "good time":

> Yes, I miss my wife. But I have a girl friend. I cut up and relax. I cut up like a kid. I have a lot more fun now than when I was married. I laugh and cut up, dance, and jog . . . My friends say, "It's your life, do with it what you may." And that's just about the way I feel about it. I can't take it with me [at this point he tries not to cry].

Then he paused and, with the sound of a dark secret in his voice, told of worrying about what the people at church were saying about his middle-aged girl friend.

And there is an odd aspect to this form of negative self-esteem. Interviewees with low self-esteem who felt cheated or betrayed sometimes appear to actually turn away from even *positive* experiences. After telling me about the importance of patience to the success of his long marriage, one of the low self-esteem interviewees paused and, with sadness in his voice, said, "If . . . a lot of good things happen to people [a long pause] . . . that is the worst thing that could happen to them." That equivocal and haunting statement seemed an unconditional resignation to a world that he had come to regard as hostile, a world in which even the *good*, in the long run, turns out *bad*.

But what if everything is too good? So good that one would choose not to change anything? There is an Arabic saying that we must be wary if things are going too well. Perhaps it goes back to the story of Polycrates, as told by the ancient Greek historian Herodotus.[6]

> Polycrates made himself king of Samos. He divided his kingdom into three parts, sharing it with his two brothers. Soon, however, he killed one brother and banished the other. He not only stole from his brothers and countrymen, but conquered one nation after another.

Kind Hearts

Herodotus wrote, "He plundered all, without distinction of friend or foe; for a friend [he said] was better pleased if you gave him back what you had taken from him, than if you spared him at the first."[7]

Then the Egyptian king, Amasis, one of Polycrates's few friends, wrote him a letter of warning. Polycrates's successes, the letter read, would provoke the envy of the gods. Better to "win some and lose some," otherwise the gods might restore the balance by taking revenge. The only way out, Amasis warned, was for Polycrates to throw away the one possession that he loved above all others.

Polycrates heeded this advice and chose what he valued most: a signet ring with an emerald set in gold. Polycrates boarded one of his ships and put out to sea. When the ship was several miles from shore, he threw the ring overboard. He breathed a sigh of relief, thinking he had ensured success without end.

Weeks later a fisherman came to the palace. He had caught a fish so large and beautiful that he thought it worthy of a king's dinner. Polycrates was delighted and invited the fisherman to join him for dinner. But when the cook cut open the fish, he found not only choice fillets, but a beautiful signet ring. Overjoyed, he took it to Polycrates. When Polycrates saw that it was the ring he had thrown away, his heart sank. Shaken, he sent a letter to Amasis telling him what had happened.

Amasis immediately dispatched a herald to Polycrates with an edict that dissolved their friendship. Polycrates, he said, had to be left to his fate, and Amasis did not want to be there when it happened.

Years later Polycrates's good fortune came to an end. He was put to death in the same manner that he had executed so many others—by crucifixion.

There is something unsettling about a life or career that is too unbalanced in the direction of success. We crave joss, but, at its best, joss is never absolute. Even those blessed with good fortune live with something in their lives that they wished was not there. This is what George Bernard Shaw had in mind after hearing the great violinist Jascha Heifetz play. He sent Heifetz a note urging him to play something badly each night before he went to bed, lest he provoke the envy of the gods and die young.

Explanatory Style

There is a correlation between optimism and high self-esteem, and, conversely, between pessimism and low self-esteem. Optimism and pessimism are learned behaviors, at least for the most part. They are behaviors that relate to *explanatory style,* a term chosen by Martin Seligman, professor of psychology at Pennsylvania State University, to describe the way that we habitually respond to ourselves when bad or unpleasant things happen to us.[8] The negative event or setback can be major or minor, important or trivial, it doesn't matter; explanatory style, like joss, is pervasive.

If, for example, I am on a diet and, at one meal, can't resist a cholesterol-laden entree and a fat-filled dessert, do I tell myself that I blew the diet for one meal, but that occasionally falling off the wagon is no big deal? Or do I tell myself that this is another example of my lack of will power, and that I have never been able to stick to anything?

The "occasionally falling off the wagon" rationale is an example of an optimistic explanatory style. I, the dieter, have experienced nothing more than a temporary lapse. The "lack of will power" rationale is an example of a pessimistic explanatory style. In that instance, I, the dieter, have reinforced a belief that I have about myself: that I lack will power and can't stick to anything. An optimistic explanatory style views the lapse as *temporary*; the pessimistic explanatory style, on the other hand, views it as *permanent* or *enduring*, a character flaw.

Seligman observed that whether one's explanatory style is optimistic or pessimistic makes a world of difference: "An optimistic explanatory style stops helplessness, whereas a pessimistic style spreads helplessness. Your way of explaining events to yourself determines how helpless you can become, or how energized, when you encounter the everyday setbacks as well as momentous defeats."[9]

Explanatory style is a habit, an acquired response, a split-second behavior that occurs before we know it. But it is also much more. "Explanatory style," Seligman says, "stems directly from your view of your place in the world—whether you think you are valuable and deserving, or worthless and hopeless. It is the hallmark of whether you are an optimist or pessimist."[10] Explanatory style has a hand-in-glove relationship to both self-esteem and joss.

Each of the heart attack survivors I interviewed had experienced disappointments and setbacks, that, at the time, must have been crushing and overwhelming. The differences between high- and low self-esteem interviewees were not in the way the disappointments and setbacks were felt at the time they were experienced, but in the feelings that remained years, even decades, later.

Disappointments and setbacks hurt, regardless of feelings of high or low self-worth. The difference is that interviewees with high self-esteem tend to remember their disappointments or setbacks as temporary, unfortunate occurrences—occurrences that they "made the best of," a phrase used by most of the high self-esteem interviewees but never by a low self-esteem interviewee. The phrase "made the best of" was usually followed by an explanation of how good can come from bad. Statements such as "made the best of it" or "good coming from bad" were never heard from the interviewees with low self-esteem.

Internalization and self-blame underscored the responses of low self-esteem interviewees to questions about the causes of their heart attacks. Unlike interviewees with high self-esteem, who named such things as high chloresterol, stress, or being overweight, low self-esteem interviewees focused on the precipitating event, often blaming themselves for setting the heart attack scenario in motion:

> I was doing volunteer work for the Red Cross just to fill the time and stay away from booze. I was delivering those plastic bags from the headquarters to the hospital . . . had to carry them from the car to the laboratory at the hospital. I mention this because *carrying those boxes had something to do with it.*

Well, *what really caused it, I think, was that I
was working around some of those trees in
the back yard,* big pine trees, and I had
worked real hard that day. I shouldn't have
been out in the yard.

I went shopping that afternoon. I know it was
carrying all those groceries from my car to my
apartment that caused the heart attack. *It was
my fault* for buying so many groceries and
trying to carry them up to my apartment.

Negative stereotyping of the aged as a group resonates to self-blame, either identifying oneself as a
member of the stigmatized group, or, more frequently,
projecting the stigma upon others. Commenting about
another elderly man who is an usher at his church, an
interviewee with low self-esteem said, "I look across the
pews at George . . . he's so damned old and senile that
he shakes the plate when he passes it . . . Christ, I hope
I die before I get like that."

In another milieu, an automobile showroom, an 80-
year-old man with high self-esteem, who regards himself as the best car salesman in Louisiana, in response to
my question about customers who may prefer a younger
salesman, said:

Sometimes when young people come in to
buy a car, I can tell that they want to be
helped by someone young, like themselves. It
doesn't upset me, because I think they look at
me like I look at the guy who's been selling

me clothes for the past thirty-five years. His tastes are so conservative that, every time I go into the store, I hope someone else will wait on me. All that those young people are doing is looking for somebody who has the same tastes that they have. It's not that they have anything against me.

I know of no better example of joss or a positive explanatory style.

Chapter 4

What We Say to Ourselves
(*Doppelganger*)

No doubt the discovery that they have grown
old causes less sadness to many people than
it did to me. But in the first place old age, in
this respect, is like death. Some men confront
them both with indifference, not because
they have more courage than others, but
because they have less imagination.

—Marcel Proust, French novelist

A *Doppelganger* is the *me* within me, the *you* within
you. It is a ghostly double of oneself that each of us carries in his or her heart. It haunts us. It is with us always.
(It is easy to understand why German sailors chose the
term Doppelganger to describe their duffel bags.) Most
of the time we are not aware of it, but at other times it
won't let us go. During awkward moments it is a cumbersome and annoying companion that we wish were
not there. In short, an embarrassment.

My Doppelganger is the *me* that I talk to when I am

alone, driving my car, or walking my dog. It is a reality within my head. Because I am talking to me, I often pay little heed to what I say. So my thoughts ramble on as though they made no difference. And that, in a nutshell, is the problem. What I say to myself can heal, make me sick, bolster my self-esteem, or break my heart.

My thoughts may be transitory; for example, I may have had a bad day, or I may not be up to par, physically. At other times, however, what I say to myself may not be transitory. It may be the *me* that I have come to believe is the true *me*. And that is the Doppelganger that has the potential to hurt me.

The Doppelganger inhabits the world of *personal myth*, the world of the heart that, as the French mathematician and philosopher Blaise Pascal wrote more than three hundred years ago, "has its reason which reason does not know."[1] By *personal myth* I mean the unique and sacred story that each of us has about his or her deepest self.

A personal myth can empower and nourish, or denigrate and demean. It can affirm our worthiness or lacerate our souls. Sam Keen says that we do not live our myths; our myths live us.[2] Keen likens a personal myth to computer technology. Each of us is born with a certain type and quality of hardware—that is, our genetic endowments. But from the time we are born, our hardware is receiving software in the form of familial ideas and expectations, traditions, gender differences, biases, etc. The result is a collection of beliefs and perceived experiences that shape, order, and direct our lives.[3]

What were you told when you were a child? That you were beautiful or ugly? Smart or dumb? An "A" student or a future dropout? If you are Catholic, were you taught to be wary of Protestants? Or, if you are a Protestant, were you told that Catholics worship the Virgin Mary and the saints instead of God and Jesus? What were you told about drinking alcohol? Or eating certain foods? That boys don't cry and only girls play with dolls?

A troublesome personal myth is easier to deny or ignore than to confront. It takes courage to disaffirm a personal myth. A personal myth is so deeply rooted that the individual is often oblivious of its presence. And for that reason its power often goes unheeded.

My family background gave me personal myths about the godlike perfection of Robert E. Lee, the unblemished heroism of Pickett's charge during the third day of the battle at Gettysburg, opinions about race, religion, government, parenting, family, dogs, cats, etc. I can choose to affirm or disaffirm any of them. Disaffirming them, however, doesn't extinguish them. They are still there. Each in its own way is a Doppelganger.

Most people are unaware of the myths they live by. Understandably, the more "bottom line" the myth is, the more it resists recognition. However, for those untroubled by faintheartedness, there are exercises that have been developed by Jean Houston (author of *The Hero and the Goddess*), Sam Keen, Stanley Krippner, (professor of psychology, Saybrook Institute, San Francisco), and others.

An exercise of Jean Houston's[4] consists of stepping backward, literally and figuratively, into time, and imagining yourself in the skin of your same-sex parent. If you are adopted, you may choose either your adoptive or biological parent. The exercise asks that you take whatever time is needed to get a sense of what it must have been like to be in that body, with that soul and personality. Is your parent the same age as you are today? If not, what age have you chosen? Why?

In the exercise, you step back from parent to grandparent, to great grandparent, to great-great grandparent—four generations. Then, as you return in time, wearing the imaginary skin of each ancestor, you ask about his or her life—its joys, sorrows, social position, belief in God, etc. Finally you return to yourself, remain quiet, and listen for a statement from within yourself. Say it aloud.

Another exercise involves outlining one's life story. It was developed by Sam Keen.[5] In Keen's workshops, he asks that each participant imagine receiving a call from a publisher asking for an autobiography. The publisher doesn't want the autobiography in final form. All that is needed is:

(a) A list of all chapters, including a descriptive heading for each, plus a one or two sentence description. (This is especially helpful in delineating transition periods.)

(b) Ten photographs, real or imagined, that you want included. Ten is the exact number needed; no more, no less. Who did you include? Who did you leave out? Where were the photos taken? At what age were you? Why that age?

(c) A floor plan of the house in which you grew up. If there were several houses, select the one that is most significant to you. What was the significance of each room? What pictures were on the wall? Were the pictures of things? Of people? Religious pictures?

(d) A working title.

The title is very important. Titles I have heard include "Dumped On," "Born to Lose," "Always Searching," "Second Best," "Born Healer," "In Transition," "Waiting to Grow Up," and "You've Come a Long Way, Baby!" Once the guiding myth is brought to consciousness, other things fall into place.

The third exercise[6] is ongoing, and requires a large piece of construction paper—say, twelve square feet. The first step is to go through magazines or brochures and cut out pictures or statements that have appeal or meaning to you. Paste them on the board. It is important to select the pictures and statements spontaneously. Also, as the weeks go by, to replace some and leave others. Note the ones you replace and what you replace them with. Are they outdoor or indoor pictures? Are they about people or places? Who? Where?

I have an unusual story to tell about this exercise. A woman, who was a former student, brought her poster to one of my workshops. She was the only participant who brought a poster. She was worried because the pictures and clippings that she had chosen alluded to the death of a young man. She has a son, and was certain that the pictures and statements were about him. I told her not to worry, that the choice of pictures and statements, no doubt, related to a transition period she was going through—the end, or death, of one part of life, and the beginning of another. I don't know if my words helped. Then, less than three months later, a young man died unexpectedly. Not her son, but Carol's and my younger son, Gus. The exercise tapped what Jung refers to as the *collective unconscious*, the unconscious that is below our personal unconscious, and shared by all of us from earliest times—people, animals, and even plants.

In telling one's life story, especially in late life, historical accuracy is unimportant. On the first page of his autobiography, C. G. Jung wrote:

> Thus it is that I have now undertaken, in my

eighty-third year, to tell my personal myth. I can only make direct statements, only "tell stories." Whether or not the stories are "true" is not the problem. The only question is whether what I tell is *my* fable, *my* truth.[7]

What counts is that the story comes from the heart, and that it is the storyteller's truth or fable. A story told from the heart links us to the universe. There is a Chasidic saying, "God created man because he loves stories."[8]

Elders have an opportunity to tell *their* stories, *their* fables, and *their* truths as part of a program called Reminiscence that takes place in Senior Centers throughout the U.S. The success of Reminiscence has been outstanding. Since personal myths are revealed through life stories, and each life story is the exclusive property of the storyteller, it is well to begin with a birth story. As each myth's hero has a birth story, so too does each of us have a story about being born that is sacred and unique.[9] With that story begins one's pilgrimage.

Hardy storytellers let their stories take them into late adulthood, perhaps even to that moment in time when they first recognized that they had grown old in the eyes of others. For some people, the awareness of growing old is memorialized by a single incident. The French author Simone de Beauvoir[10] writes of how unpleasantly her friend Marie Dormoy's age was revealed to her. A young man, deceived by her youthful figure, followed her. As he overtook her and saw her face, instead of flirting with her, he hurried on. Another example is the poignant story told by Alex Comfort, a gerontologist and biologist, of a woman in her sixties who, after making love in a Paris hotel room that had mirrors on the ceiling, chose never to make love again. French poet and playwright Paul Claudel, on the other hand, wrote with astonishing grace and optimism, "Eighty years old! No eyes left, no ears, no teeth, no legs, no wind! And when all is said and done, how astonishingly well one does without them."[11]

After receiving the Nobel prize at the age of 57, the Irish poet W. B. Yeats expressed his exasperation and anger about growing old, "Being old makes me tired and furious; I am everything that I was and indeed more, but an enemy has bound and twisted me . . . I can no longer carry out what I plan and think."[12]

Finally, essayist Stephen Butterfield's story of his father's last years:

> When he was old, I tried to introduce him to the Buddhist doctrine of emptiness; I thought it would ease any anxiety he might be having about the imminence of death. "Ultimately," I began, "you never were." "Maybe not," he said, peering over the rim of his glasses, "but I made a hell of a splash where I should have been."[13]

Age Bias

Each of us who reaches 60 has a collection of "getting old" stories. For the most part we take them in stride, turning, as Viorst says, tragedy into irony.[14] But not always. There is nothing light or funny about age bias, especially at the hands of professionals who should know better.

This is illustrated by a true story. A questionnaire was given to students when they entered medical school, and again four years later at the time of their graduation. They were asked to rank medical disciplines on the basis of personal preference. The discipline that changed least during the four years was geriatrics. For most students it began and remained in last place.[15]

A study sponsored by the AARP of 1,860 large corporations and employment agencies indicated unfair treatment to older job applicants more than 26 percent of the time.[16] Moreover, age bias is filtering downward to middle-aged people. Between 1980 and 1992 the overall unemployment rate rose from 7.1 to 7.4 percent. During the same period, the rate for unemployed middle-aged men rose from 5.0 to 11.0 percent.[17]

Age bias and age stereotyping reinforce a negative Doppelganger. And a Doppelganger run amok can bring about serious consequences for anyone. What we say to ourselves can make us sick, break our hearts, or dispirit us to the point of sabotaging the rational aspects of personality, deterring healing, and shattering a sense of well being. Kabir, a fifteenth-century mystic Sufi poet, wrote:

> Go over and over your beads, paint weird designs on your forehead, wear your hair matted, long, and ostentatious, but when deep inside you there is a loaded gun, can you have God?[18]

"When deep inside you is a loaded gun" is a metaphor for a psychological process called *rumination*, a process of obsessive analysis, usually obsessive self-analysis. The first dictionary definition for the word *rumination* is "chewing the cud." Seligman observed that:

> Ruminant animals, such as cattle, sheep, and goats, chew a cud composed of regurgitated, partially digested food—not a very appealing image of what people who ruminate do with their thoughts, but an exceedingly apt one. Rumination combined with [a] pessimistic explanatory style is the recipe for severe depression.[19]

Existentialist psychotherapist Irvin Yalom described the ruminating, self-abasing dialogue of one of his patients as a "litany [of] depression-spawned propaganda."[20]

What we choose to call it—depression-spawned

propaganda, rumination, or a negative Doppelganger—doesn't matter. The result is the same: self-abasement that tyrannizes, bullies, and eventually thwarts one's God-given inclination toward healing, wholeness, and fullness of life.

The energetic rebuttal demanded of a confrontation with a Doppelganger out of control is expressed by the German word *Auseinandersetzung*. It is a word that Jung was fond of using. It means a vigorous and vehement discussion with oneself, arguing on your own behalf as if you were Clarence Darrow or Alan Dershowitz—arguing as though your life depended on it. And well it may.

Chapter 5

Memories That Heal, Memories That Harm

Protect me from hardness of heart.
— *The Book of Common Prayer*

"It isn't much of a memory that only works backwards," the Queen remarked.
— Lewis Carroll, author of *Alice in Wonderland*

Memories have their own set of dynamics. An analogy is to compare memories of things past to an obbligato part in music—a background melody that is essential to the piece, but is not the focus of the listener's attention. In a similar way, memories weave old themes in and out, as a psychic background to the life the individual is now leading. Memories do not stabilize. They are never static. They metamorphose in ways that can enhance or diminish us.

A memory dynamic that is positive and healing draws us toward psychological and spiritual balance. In

Jungian terms, it pulls us toward wholeness. If, on the other hand, the memory dynamic is negative, it will eat the heart, as a bird of prey ate the liver of the chained Prometheus in Greek mythology.

In 1928 the Institute of Human Development at the University of California, Berkeley, began a study of the life course of children, from birth to adolescence. Parents of every third baby born in Berkeley between late 1928 and early 1929 were given the opportunity to participate. The study tracked the medical, as well as developmental, history of each child. Included in the study were periodic interviews with the parents of the children over the course of nearly two decades.

In the early 1980s, twenty-nine of the surviving female parents were interviewed by psychoanalyst Erik Erikson, art therapist Joan Erikson, and psychologist Helen Kivnick.[1] The Eriksons and Kivnick compared their findings with interview notes that had been recorded decades earlier.

Among their findings was a tendency of the women to omit issues of discontent that had been reported during the time of the initial interviews, as recorded in the data from the 1930s and 1940s. The Eriksons and Kivnick considered several possible explanations. The first was a desire for privacy. Next was the possibility that the omissions were a conscious or unconscious reshaping or manipulation of memories; in other words, the interviewees had reincorporated memories into their lives in forms that they found acceptable. For example, a woman who, decades earlier, described her husband as having few redeeming qualities, remembered him quite differently fifty years later. In her 80s she described him not as an inadequate husband and father, but someone who, in spite of his faults, "did his best for his family." He was neither the best nor worst of fathers or husbands. The woman seemed to prove what a poet once said, "One lives by memory, not by truth."

The third possibility was that ". . . these omissions [of earlier issues of discontent] reflect a lifelong process of reintegration and recasting, whereby events and circumstances that were once experienced as painful have, over the years, taken on new meanings as part of the whole life cycle. Perhaps, in addition, they indicate that, over the years, traumatic events have been put into perspective."[2]

Reshaping of memories occurs most dramatically during periods of transition. Frequently the memories relate to parents. It doesn't matter how old we are or whether our parents are living or dead, our connections to them are forever changing. At midlife, especially, we learn to accept their shortcomings as an inevitability, rather than a flaw in parenting. Viorst said, "We see how little power they had, and how little we have now, to build sturdy bridges across the gulfs which separate us . . . we learn to give thanks for even imperfect connections."[3]

In another setting, a cemetery in Greenville, Mississippi, the poet and writer William Percy reflected on much the same thing:

> While people are still alive we judge them as good or bad, condemn them as failures or praise them as successes, love them or despise them. Only when they are dead do we see them, not with charity, but with understanding. Alive they are remote, even hostile; dead, they join our circle and you see the family likeness.[4]

Percy wrote exquisitely of memories healed by time and the separation of death. But some memories persist, often involving people alive or dead, who are, or were, oblivious to the injury they caused. In homage to the chained Prometheus of Greek myth, I call these memories *vulturine* memories. Examples are:

> A 70-year-old man who had been "down on religion" for fifty-five years because of something the minister said at his father's funeral: "I vowed never to set foot in church again, and I've been true to my word."

> An 85-year-old man who, for twenty years, has lived comfortably in an expensive Florida retirement community on a pension from a Fortune 500 company: "They never gave me the recognition they gave [another former employee] and I still resent it."

A blind retiree who felt that the auto manufacturer he worked for had cheated him: "They should have given me a car. Cars are what I built and I deserve one, even though I'm blind."

An 83-year-old man, eighteen years retired from a large insurance company, told of the hurt he still feels because of not having been included in a group of fellow employees who had lunch together each day. Most of the luncheon group had long since died, but his anger persisted. His wife interrupted to remind him that somebody had to be at the office during the noon hour, and that his co-workers had nothing against him. He responded by saying, "It doesn't matter, they didn't ask me."

Both sad and disconcerting are the thwarted efforts toward healing and forgiveness that seem to go hand in glove with vulturine memories. For example, the man who was excluded from the luncheon group said that "in spite of it all" he had "forgiven" his fellow workers. Another interviewee, a man in his mid-70s, held back tears as he complained about the inequity of his divorce settlement. He looked at me plaintively and said, "I forgive her for what she got away with."

"Eating your heart out" is more than a cliche. Several studies relate anger and hostility to heart disease. "Evidence that anger plays an important role in the development of heart disease continues to grow

. . . studies have shown that tendencies toward hostility are associated with a higher risk of dying from heart disease, and that the risk of a heart attack more than doubles in the two hours after an episode of anger."[5] Hostility is frequently linked to the onset of heart disease. It has been identified as a Type A (heart attack prone) characteristic.

The Greeks honored the power of memory. One of Zeus's wives is Mnemosyne, a goddess whose name translates to Memory. The daughters of Zeus and Memory, in classical as well as romantic literature, are known as the nine Muses. Perhaps it was to balance out Memory's double-edged gift of not forgetting, that Greek myth also includes the river Lethe. Lethe is the river of forgetfulness or oblivion, the river that separates the living world from Hades. All that was needed to forget was to drink a single drop of its water.

After talking to my students about the importance of healing bad memories and letting go of anger, a woman in her mid-30s raised her hand. She said that she felt guilty because she could not *forgive* the drunk driver who killed her husband. She was pregnant at the time, and the death of her husband left her no choice but to move in with her alcoholic mother. Her comfortable middle class life was shattered. Like her mother she became a recipient of welfare.

Jesus taught forgiveness. He also taught us to simply

"let go" of hostility and anger, however righteous, during times when contrition on the part of the perpetrator,
followed by forgiveness on the part of the victim, seem
out of the question:

> You have learned how it was said: *Eye for eye
> and tooth for tooth*. But I say this to you: offer
> the wicked man no resistance. On the con-
> trary, if anyone hits you on the right cheek,
> offer him the other as well; if a man takes you
> to law and would have your tunic, let him
> have your cloak as well. And if anyone orders
> you to go one mile, go two miles with him.[6]

More to the point are the instructions that Jesus gave
to his apostles as they set out on their missionary work:
"If they persecute you in one town, take refuge in the
next; and if they persecute you in that, take refuge in
another."[7] Jesus could not have been more explicit
about "letting go" and "putting the past behind us"
when confrontation is useless, restitution is out of the
question, and festering anger is the only alternative.

Dennis Linn and Matthew Linn, Jesuit priests, have
done an impressive amount of work on memories. The
Linns treat a bad memory as a grief to be healed. They
follow the stages of grief identified by the Swiss psychiatrist Elizabeth Kubler-Ross: denial, anger, bargaining,
depression, and resignation. Each stage is worked
through, treating the memory as a personal loss, a loss
to be mourned and healed.[8]

A not-too-serious example: What if a student or someone else who has attended one of my lectures says, "What a bore; a *phudnik* if ever I heard one." This comment upsets me because it is made by someone I admire. More disturbing, a *phudnik* is a *nudnik* with a Ph.D., and a *nudnik* is Yiddish for an insufferable bore. I feel doubly wronged. I can't shrug it off, because the person who made this comment is very intelligent. Moreover, she first heard the expressions *nudnik* and *phudnik* from me. Instead of giving way to feelings of pique, or confronting her, I decided to "let go" by going through the Kubler-Ross stages:

> 1. Denial: Obviously she meant someone else. More than likely I was being compared favorably to another teacher who is known to be pompous, loud, and pedantic—a man who is truly a bore.
>
> 2. Anger: She meant me. Now I realize that she isn't as intelligent as I thought. Like other "average" students, she wants to be spoon-fed.
>
> 3. Bargaining: From now on I will use fewer quotes, cover less material, and speak more to the point. If I do that faithfully, I will never again be called a *phudnik*.
>
> 4. Depression: Have I lost my knack? Everything has to come to an end. I enjoyed teaching and lecturing, but it may be time to retire.

5. Resignation/Acceptance: This sort of thing happens. It doesn't happen often, but it still hurts. The listener is intelligent, not average. Her comment put me back on track. Yes, at times, I am a *phudnik*, and that is something I must be careful about. All in all, however, I'm good at what I do. Now, thanks to her comment, which I didn't want to acknowledge, I'm even better.

Hurtful feelings are one thing. But what about memories of a different sort? Gut-wrenching memories? Spitting-mad memories? Memories that resonate to the anguish of the Psalmist as he cries out to Yahweh to wreak vengeance upon his enemies:

Let the table before them be a trap and their sacred
    feasts a snare.
Let their eyes be darkened, that they may not see, and
    give them continual trembling in their loins.
Pour out your indignation upon them, and let the fierce-
    ness of your anger overtake them.
Let them be wiped out of the book of the living and not
    be written among the righteous.[9]

I have no answer for this kind of anger in late adulthood or any other time of life, other than that such hostility, if not dealt with, harms us in every way—body, mind, and soul. Perhaps it is enough that that Psalm— usually without the verses above—is often paired in the

Lectionary of Christian churches with the passage from Matthew, also quoted above, "If they persecute you in one town, take refuge in the next; and if they persecute you in that, take refuge in another."

If a more prestigious authority on the importance of the healing of memories is needed, few are more compelling than Pope John Paul II. John Paul refers to the healing of memories as the call of reconciliation, and says that it is the most important task that confronts our elders:

> As you look on your lives you may remember sufferings and personal failures. It is important to think about these experiences, so as to see them in the light of the whole life's journey. You may realize that some events which brought you suffering also brought you many blessings . . . As Christians we *should offer our memories to the Lord.* Thinking about the past will not alter the reality of your sufferings or disappointments, but it can change the way you look at them . . . And when it is done in prayer it can be a source of healing.[10]

Chapter 6

Trust and the Loss of Self-Reliance

There are good men everywhere, at all times.
Most men are. Some are just unlucky,
because men are a little better than their circumstances give them a chance to be. And
I've known some that even the circumstances
couldn't stop.

—William Faulkner, Southern
writer

If the aspect of growing old that most haunts us were to
be singled out, it most likely would be the fear of
becoming dependent upon others. The thought of rely-
ing on someone else to do those things that we take for
granted—preparing meals, shopping, even getting out
of bed—evokes fear the world over. But in no other culture is that fear as great as among older Americans.

That fear brings to mind my visit to a retirement
community located in the Midwest. The owners of the
retirement community had proudly purchased dozens
of rocking chairs. They were handsome rockers, and
they had been placed throughout the building. There

were rockers in the lobby, on the front porch, even in alcoves along the hallways. To the owners' surprise, many of the residents refused to sit in them; some, with great physical effort, retrieved chairs from their apartments or from storage rooms, placed them next to the rockers, and sat in silent protest. The connotations of a rocking chair—frailty, helplessness, and dependency— were not to be tolerated by this group of elders. True bloody-mindedness!

The French journalist Alexis de Tocqueville, whose observations of early-nineteenth-century America form the basis of much of our social history, singled out self-sufficiency as an American characteristic, but he did not praise it. "Thus not only does democracy make every man forget his ancestors, but it hides his descendants and separates his contemporaries from him; it throws him back forever upon himself alone, and threatens in the end to confine him entirely within the solitude of his own heart."[1]

Ralph Waldo Emerson, whose truths have inspired us for more than a century, carried de Tocqueville's observations a step further. He defined discontent as "the want of self-reliance" and an "infirmity of will."[2]

After extensive interviews with middle- to upper-income retirees living in Los Angeles and Santa Barbara, a research firm reported that, next to moving to a nursing home, the greatest fear of the people interviewed was the fear of becoming a burden to their children,

Kind Hearts

especially having to move in with them.[3] At the time of the study, America was in a recession, and memories of the Great Depression were easily stirred; many of the interviewees recalled the disruptive experience of three-generation families that had been forced to live together. The findings of the marketing firm were in line with the need for maintaining a sense of control of one's life, which is a hallmark of social gerontology.

Still, self-reliance has its limits. A recent study hypothesized that overall self-sufficiency among elderly women, including an ability to perform tasks that are normally performed by males, would predict life satisfaction.[4] This turned out not to be so, at least not to the extent the researcher expected. Although generally true, the correlation between self-sufficiency and life satisfaction was not absolute. Instead, life satisfaction was highest among widows whose circumstances were characterized by a minimal degree of dependency. This group of women experienced less loneliness than those who thought of themselves as totally self-sufficient. The minimally dependent widows felt loved by those upon whom they relied; their feelings of high self-worth mirrored the way they saw themselves in the eyes of others.[5]

No one wants to give up his or her independence. Nor do we wish such losses on our parents or anyone else. However, such losses are not always totally bad or catastrophic. As Martin Luther, the leader of the

German Reformation, said almost five hundred years ago, "God works in contraries, at times bestowing blessings where most people see only an ordeal." Such was the experience of Stephen Butterfield in caring for his father:

> After he turned senile, I did not like taking on the responsibility for his care. . . . sometimes I wished him a speedy death. Now I can see how his long period of decline gave me a chance to feel close to him again. I needed that chance, in order to dissolve any lingering vestiges of alienation from myself. . . . Alzheimer's disease gradually took all the battles out of him. In the end, he was as gentle as a toothless old cat, smiling and weak, fumbling with his chain. I did not resent him for anything. Whatever had divided us came unwound, along with the connections of his brain.[6]

Trust is a gift of late adulthood. It is also a gift to the newborn. Basic trust is learned during the first year of life. It is the developmental task upon which all other tasks learned over a lifetime are to be built.

Much later, at midlife, trust emerges once again. This time it is a part of what Erikson termed *generativity,*[7] the next-to-last psychosocial stage. Generativity affirms a sense of trust in the next generation. It means stepping back, so to speak, and letting those who are younger and less experienced have their turn. Generativity affirms the sacredness and correctness of the cycle of life, death, and rebirth (or renewal).

The cycle of life, death, and rebirth is most beautifully expressed in the Elusinian mysteries of ancient Greece, which were performed annually to celebrate the harvest and to memorialize the story of Demeter and Persephone.

In that myth, Demeter searched all the earth, looking for Persephone, her lost daughter. She discovered that Persephone had been ravished by Hades, god of the underworld, and taken to the world of the dead. Demeter's grief was unending. She was the goddess of agriculture, and, since each immortal expressed rage in ways appropriate to his or her mythic role, Demeter kept all the corn on earth from growing. Zeus intervened, and Persephone was allowed to leave Hades and return to her mother, but her return was conditional. She had eaten some seeds of a pomegranate, a fruit that symbolized fecundity and came from the blood of Dionysus. In atonement, Persephone was forced to return to the land of the dead for a period of six months each year. Thus the cycle of the seasons, of planting and harvesting, of death and rebirth.

Demeter's sorrow has a haunting application to the sorrow that comes to some of our elders in advanced old age. Losses ranging from physical attractiveness, agility of mind, sexuality, and social status cause some of our elders to silently rage against the inevitable, just as Demeter raged over the loss of Persephone.[8] To these individuals, trust, if it comes at all, comes with difficulty and great pain.

To others, the experience is quite different, although their losses may be equally painful. Instead of anguishing over the inevitability of losses that can never be recovered, these exceptional people seem to grow rather than diminish in spirit. Paradoxically, this *still point* seems less related to promises of a life to come than to an acceptance of life as one has chosen to live it.

Jungian analyst Robert Johnson[9] makes this point in his interpretation of the myth of Psyche and Eros, although he does not speak of trust as being central to the heroine's journey. However, it is implied throughout. In the myth, Psyche and Eros are lovers that live in an orgasmic paradise. Eros works away from home all day. His job is shooting love darts at anyone he happens to see.

Eros returns home each evening and spends the night with Psyche. They are superb lovers and truly happy, except in one respect: Psyche has promised never to look upon Eros's face. It is, of course, a promise meant to be broken, and that is exactly what Psyche does. Beautiful but something of a klutz, she is urged by her sisters to look upon Eros's face. She does and falls even more deeply in love with him. But in the rapture of viewing his face, she knocks over a lamp and spills oil on him. He awakens, throws a tantrum, and, in a childish pique, goes home to his mother, Aphrodite. To win Eros back, Psyche agrees to perform four tasks that are contrived by Aphrodite.

Each task seems outrageous and impossible to complete. The first is for Psyche to sort a huge mound of seeds. She faints. The task is accomplished by ants who come to her rescue while she sleeps. Next she must bring Aphrodite the golden fleece of a ram, a challenge that has claimed the lives of many brave men. Psyche is again saved by the unexpected: a "talking" reed growing from a pond. It tells her to wait until dusk, cross the river, and retrieve strands of golden fleece that were pulled from the coat of a ram as it thrashed through brambles. Only a small amount of fleece is needed. She *trusts* the reed and retrieves the golden fleece. (The need for only a small amount of fleece has a late-midlife characteristic. In fairy tales about midlife we are told to take nothing more into late life than what is truly needed.[10] We must trust that it will be enough.)

Psyche's third task is to fill a goblet with water from a raging river, without spilling the water or shattering the goblet on the rocks below. She *entrusts* the task to an eagle. Here, the water and goblet are analogous to psychotherapy. The goblet keeps the water (psychic content) from spilling out and injuring the client, and sometimes the therapist as well.

To complete the fourth task, Psyche must *trust* in the

wisdom of a "talking" tower. That task is to journey into Hades and retrieve a vial of perfume that is coveted by Aphrodite. The tower tells her that, to complete this task, she must learn to *say no*. But not simply saying no to trivial requests; she must say no to people in dire circumstances. Psyche's no is the *creative no*, which is essential to protecting our energies from demands that stifle and destroy.

Psyche enters the world of the dead and returns with the vial of perfume. She almost bungles again by using some of the perfume herself. Eros, however, comes to her rescue. The lovers are reunited and permitted to live forever in the world of the gods.

Trust is part and parcel of creativity, and the nature of the feminine is to create. This, says Joseph Wheelwright, a Jungian analyst and founder of the C. G. Jung Institute of San Francisco, is because women give birth, create life, and "confront life and death in ways men will never know."[11] The Psyche and Eros legend speaks to both the masculine and feminine, but more to the feminine.

The "going home" stories—stories about the return of the conquering Greeks from the Trojan War—are about trust, creativity, and the masculine journey to the feminine. Of the Greek heroes, however, only Odysseus completes the journey in every sense of the word. The other Greek heroes do not fare as well. Some fare quite badly: Agamemnon is murdered by his wife and her lover. Menelaus settles down to what must have been an edgy household with Helen, his unfaithful wife, whose adulterous affair started the ten years of bloody warfare. Only Odysseus completes the adventure at a psychic as well as a physical level.

All of Odysseus's lessons, including trust, are learned from women. The sorceress Circe, for example, tells him that if he is to successfully navigate between Scylla and Charybdis (the monster and the whirlpool that have come to symbolize impossible choices in life), he must not resist the dangers he will confront.[12] He must ride them out. Instead, he girds his armor, paying no attention to Circe's admonition and its deeper meaning that his time for heroism is over. His ship is destroyed and he almost loses his life.

Finally, after years of struggle, with his ships destroyed and his crew and soldiers dead, Odysseus is washed ashore from the sea (which symbolizes the unconscious). Nausicaa, a beautiful nubile princess, finds him and he is, at last, returned home. Odysseus, whose feminine self may be represented by Nausicaa, has received, among the other gifts of wholeness, the gift of learning to trust.

For many of us, the odyssey or pilgrimage that teaches us to trust and, as Wheelwright[13] says, "learn to live in the deep," comes from a life-threatening illness, an illness that tries the soul as well as the body. As Rachel

Naomi Remen observed, the words *cancer* or *heart attack*, words that connote suffering and death, turn us into seekers and command us to discard pretense.[14]

Remen likened this inner search to restoring an old house that is filled with shabby and frayed furniture. As the old furniture and clutter are thrown away, or put in a box to give to charity, an inner voice keeps saying, "Wait, that's a perfectly good lamp," or "Maybe I can use that old chair somewhere?" Perhaps so. It may be a perfectly good lamp and the old chair may come in handy some day. But that isn't the point. The point is that the lamp has to go. The chair, too. Everything that isn't *you* has to go. It may hurt, but there is no going back.

Albert Kreinheder, director emeritus of the C. G. Jung Institute of Los Angeles, in a small and heroic book written just prior to his death, said that to do away with pretense is to confront truth as though truth itself carried the image of God.

> There is one guideline that is more important than any others, and that is truth. We have to be totally and completely truthful with ourselves. So-called positive thinking is a pale, sentimental sort of thing if it is just a covering over of reality. The soul does not thrive on deceit. Truth is the elixir. Truth is the panacea. Truth is the most precious of psychic ingredients, and it is almost a synonym for God.[15]

Kind Hearts

Chapter 7

Money and Self-Esteem

Her voice is full of money, he said suddenly. That was it. I'd never understood before. It was full of money—that was the inexhaustible charm that rose and fell in it . . . High in a white palace the king's daughter, the golden girl.

—F. Scott Fitzgerald, American novelist

The love of money as a possession—as distinguished from the love of money as a means to the enjoyment and realities of life—will be recognized for what it is, a somewhat disgusting morbidity, one of those semi-criminal, semi-pathological propensities which one hands over with a shudder to the specialists in mental disease.

—John Maynard Keynes, English economist

He was . . . subject to a kind of disease, which at that time they called lack of money.

—Rabelais, French satirist

Rabelais is close to the mark. A lack of money can be dispiriting to the point of seeming like a disease. So, too, is the thought of not having enough money to meet future needs. This dread, which is omnipresent in many of our elders, occurs in many ways: the threat of rising health-care costs, increases in the cost of living, the possibility of outliving one's source of income, etc.

This chapter, however, is not about money per se. It is, instead, about the intrapsychic meaning of money as it relates to the presence or absence of feelings of self-worth.

When I began to study elderly heart attack survivors, it did not occur to me to probe for perceptions of money. I did not think money was an issue. The interviewees lived in relatively expensive homes and, based on appearances, seemed well off. There was also another, more practical, reason. I did not want them to refuse to answer a question, midway during the interviews, just because I asked them about something they didn't want to talk about. So the subject of money came up without probing on my part.

But first a personal note. I once felt ill at ease, or more accurately queasy, when talking about money. Why this was so, I had not the foggiest notion. I did know that not being able to talk about money had raised havoc with many aspects of my life, ranging from marriage to business ventures. Oddly, I had no problem talking with bankers about commercial real estate loans. However, I could not deal with wage or commission complaints. Nor could I collect fees owed to me without feeling awkward, sometimes even embarrassed. Worse, I was convinced that my attitudes toward money were not only unusual but, probably, unique. So I did what people trained in psychology do—I sought help from a psychotherapist. Through her skills I quickly identified the source of my problem, and in one brief session my awkwardness was resolved. Now I know how to talk about money. Still, from time to time, I have to repeat the exercises the therapist taught me.

This anecdote is included for two reasons. First, because I know personally about the mythic, intrapsychic, properties of money, and the harm they can cause. If there is doubt about money having psychic energy, read the libretto of Wagner's *Der Ring des Nibelungen* in which the principal characters, Alberich, the Nibelung, and Wotan, the highest mythic god, struggle with greed, avarice, and a lust for power. Or, in modern terms, the misuse of money.

The second reason is that there is *no* normal attitude about money. (It is easier to define a normal attitude about sex.) Still, the energy of money is pervasive, and it influences almost all parts of life: marriage, friendship, education, and even religion. Notice the congregation at church the next time money is talked about. Is there the same dynamic when a new theological idea is proposed? Which causes more people to look about, aimlessly and nervously? Or more people to squirm in the pews?

Two people can be friends for years until one asks the other for a loan. Except among students or theatrical people, where borrowing back and forth is a way of life, the friendship will never be the same.

Books about money have been published without end. Each year brings new titles ranging from acquiring "riches without effort" to "forgetting about money and letting a windfall happen." None, however, touched upon money intrapsychically until Jacob Needleman's *Money and the Meaning of Life*.

Needleman is not a professor of business. I am almost certain that he is not an MBA. His field is philosophy. In writing about the intrapsychic properties of money, he is pioneering new ground. Needleman builds upon the well-known passage from St. Matthew in which the Pharisees attempt to ensnare Jesus with a question about monetary tributes to Caesar. Jesus said:

> Render therefore unto Caesar the things which are Caesar's; and unto God the things that are God's.

The next verse reads:

> When they had heard these words, they marveled, and left him, and went their way.[1]

The first verse is central to Needleman's work. In

essence, it is the importance of being able to live life at two levels, the spiritual and the material. The second verse tells us that Jesus's response is more important than first meets the eye. The Pharisees, who seldom marveled openly at anything Jesus said or did, marveled at that statement.

Marveled is the word chosen in the King James Version. Other translators use other words or phrases. Regardless, it was not simply a quick and pithy rejoinder on Jesus's part. Instead it encapsulates one of the consuming tasks of life: the task of separating that which is God's, the spiritual, from that which is Caesar's, the material—and, most importantly, honoring both.

> The making of money, the accumulation of material goods, draws man to trust too much in the lower nature of his well-being. It draws us to give it first place. At the same time, *the lower nature has a place*, and a very strong place. The need for material well-being arises out of the transitory, but *real*, lower nature of man. And so the challenge of human life is that of rendering unto Caesar that which is Caesar's—*no more and no less*—and unto God that which is God's—*no more and no less*. The challenge is to live a two-natured life, according to the unique ontological structure of the human creature.[2]

Needleman views money as "an instrument in the search for self-knowledge."[3] and, as such, an instrument that is sensitive to feelings of self-worth.

Examples of this quality are seen in Shelly Taylor's[4] study of women with breast cancer and in my[5] work with elderly heart attack survivors. Taylor observed three characteristics that were present in those women whose recoveries from breast cancer were most successful. The first was a sense of mastery over a recurrence. Each successful survivor had done something to protect herself from a recurrence: for example, changing a life-style or giving up smoking.

The second characteristic was a favorable comparison with others. Taylor's study involved younger women, but a favorable comparison with others is also indicative of a healthy and positive self-concept in late life. Elders who rate their health as good usually compare themselves favorably to their contemporaries. They also think of themselves as appearing and acting younger than others of the same age.

The third characteristic, and the most interesting of the three, consisted of each successful survivor doing something special for herself. Often it involved spending money in ways that, under other circumstances, may have been thought of as self-indulgent or extravagant. Here, however, that which appeared extravagant or self-indulgent was, in fact, a sound and sensible statement of self-worth.

In my interviews of heart attack survivors with high self-esteem, similar stories of self-affirmation emerged:

My wife and I took a trip out west to the Badlands. It was something I always wanted to do, but kept putting it off until I got the money. After my heart attack I decided not to wait.

I traded in my year-old Cadillac for a new one. Normally, I'd have waited a couple of years.

At first blush, both comments seem fatalistic, and in a way they are. But looked at in another way, each comment ritualizes the sacredness of the individual's life. Not a memorial, but an act of celebration, the way that crowds gather in Key West each day at sunset to applaud the day that has been. These self-affirmations give, perhaps, a new and more insightful understanding to architect Frank Lloyd Wright's comment that, if he could have the luxuries of life, he would willingly do without the necessities.[6]

Among the heart attack interviewees, there were no differences in frugality or generosity between people with high or low self-esteem. The differences were in their perceptions of money. Persons with low self-esteem talked about clever investments and, in two interviews, the skills by which they managed to prosper to the disadvantage of others. Others talked about influencing the behavior of their children or grandchildren by granting or withholding money. Their stories were reminiscent of psychologist David Gutmann's seminal cross-cultural studies of the stereotypical old man as power broker:[7] for example, the old man in primal societies who controlled land, wealth, and women, and granted them to younger men at his whim.

People with high self-esteem did not talk about money as instruments of power. Money was talked about in a broader context:

> I haven't made a lot of money but I've never been in a bind.

> The Lord always knew how much money I could handle.

> If I want something, or if the grandchildren want something, I buy it . . . if I can't afford it I ask to pay later . . . if they say "no" I figure we don't need it.

In no instance did an interviewee with high self-esteem speak of using money shrewdly or as a means to control another person. There are, of course, no absolutes. It would be difficult to imagine having money and not, from time to time, misusing its power. Thereby confusing, so to speak, God and Caesar.

Chapter 8

Disengaging Gently

My dear Macintosh:

The main practical thing for you to remember is that you are now sixty-five and on the point of retirement. For heaven's sake, retire and do not persuade yourself that you are a special case. If you have kept mind and body active, a world of new interest lies before you. If not, then you have no business to cling to office, or indeed to any voluntary or other service to which you are attached. Clear out. Do not rationalize by saying that you "want to see this thing through." That is just another barnacle argument; what you really want to do is to cling.

> —Professor James M.
> Macintosh, from a letter to
> himself, written when he was
> 42 years old, and opened on
> his 65th birthday.

In 1965 I presented my first paper about aging. It was presented in Los Angeles at the eighteenth annual meeting of the Gerontological Society of America. The paper was an amateurish effort. To this day, I wonder at the chutzpa of me as a young man with little background, academic or applied, telling America's premier gerontologists that providing an opportunity for purposeful activities to an older population would result in enhanced vigor, a higher quality of life, and perhaps even a longer life. One of the ranking members told me afterward that the absence of applause—there had been dead silence—was because I was "flying in the face of the leading theory of the day: disengagement."[1] I was not "torn apart," he said, only because I was too young to know better.

I still feel a twinge each time the word *disengagement* appears in a book I am reading. And since relatively few books on gerontology omit a section on disengagement, I feel that twinge quite often. In essence, disengagement theory says that in late adulthood we withdraw (disengage) from activities, work-related as well as social, that have been important and meaningful to us. Sometimes the disengagement is gradual. At other times, as in retirement, it comes all at once. The second part of the theory is that not only do we choose to disengage, but our environment and the people in it encourage us to do so.[2]

If disengagement goes smoothly, chances are that the transition to late adulthood and all that it implies will be relatively easy. More important, the individual's quality of life will be relatively high. By the same token, if we cling and resist instead of disengaging willingly, the transition to, and the experience of, late adulthood will be less than satisfactory.

Not more than a few years after my fiasco in Los Angeles, the prevailing gerontological view shifted from disengagement to *activity theory*. Activity theory suggests that "older people who are aging optimally stay active and resist shrinkage in their social world."[3] In other words, our elders, who are aging optimally, continue the activities of midlife and find substitutes for any activity that has to be given up.

Gerontology, it seemed, had found a new and more palatable paradigm. I supported it enthusiastically. I still do. But not to the exclusion of disengagement—or, more accurately, partial disengagement. By partial disengagement I refer to a recognition and acceptance of some, but not all, of the restrictions of growing older that are part of normal aging.

On a personal note:

> I no longer take late-night airplane flights and search for hotels in unfamiliar cities, going to bed at 2:00 a.m. and getting up at 7:00 or 8:00 a.m. (It was always unpleasant.)

> I no longer play singles tennis, and my doubles game is not what it used to be. (Since starting this book, my doubles game has gone, too.)

I avoid driving at night if at all possible.

I no longer run for airplanes, arriving at the airport minutes before departure time.

I avoid "working" dinners, lunches, and early morning breakfast meetings.

I do not feel compelled to read all the books people lend me, however benign their intentions.

Leaving tasks undone until tomorrow or the next day doesn't bother me. (In truth it never did.) I cherish the depth of the Yiddish admonition, "What difference does it make if the Messiah comes an hour later?"

By the same token:

I work as enthusiastically now as I did when I was younger. But I do not work as long, and when I feel tired I stop.

I still get goose flesh when I hear Brahms or Mahler, I still fall in love with Ingrid Bergman each time I see *Casablanca*, and I am still ready to abandon good sense each time I hear the Prelude to Wagner's *Tristan und Isolde*.

The list is almost without end. What is important is that I miss none of the things I disengaged from. I shudder at the thought of playing singles tennis with a 30 to

40-year-old. Running for airplanes was never pleasant. And unless I decide to go to bed at nine or ten every night, breakfast meetings don't make sense.

To *partially* disengage means to let go of some, but *not all*, of the activities that once were important. It means easing up on others. It also means replacing some of those activities with new activities.

Each of the heart attack survivors I interviewed felt that his or her coronary had narrowed available options. None, however, had to rely on others for necessities such as shopping, visiting friends, or going to church. The narrowing of options pertained rather to leisure activities that they once enjoyed without restriction.

Gardening was frequently mentioned. Those who enjoyed gardening found it more tiring than before their heart attacks. The difference was that people with low self-esteem tended to give it up altogether. Those with high self-esteem did not. The high self-esteem gardeners simply worked at it more leisurely, and only when they felt like it. A man with low self-esteem said:

> On a little place like this I have to get a yard man to do the yard . . . I fatigue easily. I enjoyed gardening and the yard, but I can't do that type of work anymore . . . it makes me so sad. I look out the front window and want to cry.

A man with high self-esteem focused on the pleasures of gardening rather than in the quality of his work.

> Sometimes, working in the garden, I have shortness of breath. If I do, I go off and do something less tiring or rest . . . then go back to gardening later . . . or do it tomorrow. You learn to do things with a little more moderation.

A civilized example of disengaging, also involving gardening, is that chosen by a gardening club of elderly Southern ladies. They meet monthly at a private club, enjoy superb food, and socialize in elegant surroundings. The president of the gardening club said, "Most of us gave up gardening years ago. This club is for drinking, eating, and dancing."

Interviewees with high self-esteem tended to disengage partially. In no instance was there a sense of urgency or a feeling of thwarted ambition:

> I just analyzed it. I've always cut my lawn, taken care of the house, and so forth. But I'd be a fool to try to keep up the same pace now. I trim the shrubbery . . . fiddle around a little bit until I get tired. Then I quit. I got me a contractor for my lawn. The house needed painting, so I got a painter.

> I like to design and build things [referring to his ham radio set] but I have a hard time getting parts. So I poke along from day to day and wait for what's going to happen tomorrow.

I slowed down some 'cause I had to. I take my time. If I get things done, all right! If I don't, I don't care! I used to want to get things done today. That was before the heart attack. Not now, though. You can't rush things if you want to do them right.

I'm a carpenter and I work on my own, so I don't have to report to anybody. It takes longer to do the work. Sometimes twice as long. But I think the quality may be a little better.

Some of your goals change as you get to retirement age . . . some of them you haven't reached. All my life I wanted to own my own business, and just before retirement I got an offer that would have made that possible. I considered it seriously, but I was too near retirement age. I figured that I would just be getting established when I wanted to retire. For reasons like that, you might change goals . . . It's not that I didn't like the work, I just wanted the time.

There are things I'd like to do, but I can't afford to hire somebody to come here [to help care for his invalid wife] . . . places I'd like to go. But I say, "That's how it is; what are you going to do?" Maybe I'm a fatalist. I think this is the worst town in America. If my wife's relatives weren't living nearby, I'd move. How do I maintain a positive attitude. Hell, it's just me . . . I was always that way. I just make the best of it. Every day is different, you know. I don't say that I don't blow my stack now and then. If I didn't, the guys in the white coats would be out there waiting for me. My philosophy is that you accept life as it comes along, and don't worry about it.

Two women from the heart attack survivor group who had low self-esteem complained that their maids did not perform to their standards. They were apologetic about the way their houses looked. On the other hand, a woman with high self-esteem said that her housekeeper did not clean as well as she would like, but that she was happy to have someone else to do the work.

In fairy tales about midlife, disengagement is a constant theme. Tales that appeared over a span of hundreds of years, from opposite ends of the world, repeatedly tell us to disengage, to let go of pretense, to withdraw projections of status, and, most important, to take no more than what is needed into old age.[4] These losses, the fairy tales tells us, are replaced with inner treasures. Sidonie Gabrielle Colette, the French novelist, wisely observed, "It is the image in the mind that binds us to our lost treasures, but it is the loss that shapes the image."[5]

This chapter began with an excerpt from a letter written by Professor Macintosh to himself when he was 42 years old. It is appropriate to conclude with Macintosh's answer to himself, written at the age of 65:

My dear Macintosh:

Many thanks for your letter of twenty-three years ago. I opened it, as you directed, on my sixty-fifth birthday. A little solemn, I thought—but then you were addressing a man old enough to be your father.

The plain truth is that I must not make a virtue out of necessity: I retire at sixty-five and that's that. I am not a special case. Thanks all the same for your friendly advice, which I shall try humbly to follow. It has been such fun since you wrote . . .

Yours truly,

—Professor James M. Macintosh[6]

Chapter 9

No One Blushes Alone

Just as no one blushes alone, so too the internal vascular system—including blood pressure, heart rate, and blood flow—is highly
responsive to human interaction.

—James J. Lynch, M.D.

Heart disease is a disease of loneliness. It is a
disease of isolation.

—Bruno Cortis, M.D., a
cardiologist

It is in the shelter of each other that people
live.

—Irish proverb

This chapter is about loneliness. Much of it is inspired
by the work and findings of Dr. James J. Lynch of the
University of Maryland School of Medicine. Lynch's two
books, *The Broken Heart* and *Language of the Heart*,
are about loneliness and the body's response to human
dialogue. Both should be required reading for anyone
who works in the field of applied gerontology, and kept

at hand for those of us who have crossed, or are about to cross, the age threshold into late adulthood.

After an exhaustive study of the cardiovascular reactions of people from a wide variety of backgrounds who were experiencing varying types of stress, ranging from divorce to accident trauma, Lynch summarizes the central thesis of his book: "The lack of human companionship, the sudden loss of love, and chronic human loneliness are significant contributors to serious disease (including cardiovascular disease) and premature death."[1]

Loneliness kills. And each time we read or hear of one of our elders who died alone and was not found until days later, we can presume that that death involved a broken heart, metaphorically if not literally.

Loneliness can come upon us at any age. But somehow in late adulthood it comes in spades: the loss of friends, the loss of a spouse, etc. More horrifying, the loss of oneself through dementias such as stroke or Alzheimer's disease.

Sometimes loneliness has nothing to do with the presence or absence of other people. Sadly, the presence of others—even, or perhaps especially, family— can intensify loneliness. The American writer Thomas Wolfe wrote, "Which of us has known his brother? Which of us has looked into his father's heart? Which of us has not remained forever prisonpent? Which of us is not forever a stranger and alone?"[2]

Most painful of all is the psychic separation that accompanies illnesses such as stroke or Alzheimer's disease. The poet Andrew Hudgens wrote about the anguish, frustration, and love of a daughter caring for her senile father, and trying at the same time to hold family and household together:

> Who knows? One glory of a family is you'd never choose your kin and can't unchoose your daddy's hazel eyes—no more than you could unchoose your hand. You get to be, in turn, someone you'd never choose to be.[3]

The strength of such human bonding inspired awe and wonderment in the nineteenth-century philosopher Arthur Schopenhauer:

> How is it that a human being can so participate in the peril and pain of another that without thought, spontaneously, he sacrifices his own life to the other? How can it happen that what we normally think of as the first law of nature and self-preservation is suddenly dissolved?

Schopenhauer's answer is that:

> . . . such a psychological crisis represents the breakthrough of a metaphysical realization, which is that you and the other are one, that you are two aspects of the one life, and that your apparent separateness is but an effect of the way we experience forms under

Kind Hearts

the conditions of space and time.[4]

The English poet and clergyman John Donne, two hundred years before Schopenhauer, said much the same thing:

> No man is an island, entire of itself . . . any man's death diminishes me, because I am involved in mankind; and therefore never send to know for whom the bell tolls; it tolls for thee.[5]

Also, in the Book of Genesis we are told of the passengers of the ark:

> That very day Noah and his sons . . . boarded the ark, with Noah's wife and the three wives of his sons, and with them wild beasts of every kind, cattle of every kind, reptiles of every kind that crawls on the earth, birds of every kind, all that flies, everything with wings. One pair of all that is flesh and has the breath of life boarded the ark with Noah; and so there went in a male and female of every creature that is flesh, just as God had ordered him. *And Yahweh closed the door behind Noah.*[6]

The last sentence, which Father Richard Rohr interprets, "And God *locked* the door behind Noah," sums it up.[7] We are closed in, not only with each other, but with all the creatures of the world—beautiful, slimy, repulsive, untouchable, exquisite—whether we like it or not. And, finally, from the Bible, the most basic tenet of all, "Yahweh God said, 'It is not good that the man should be alone. I will make him a helpmate.'"[8]

Loneliness predisposes us to disease, especially heart disease. Dr. Leonard Syme,[9] epidemiologist, University of California, Berkeley, ranks loneliness as a risk factor just as important as smoking, high cholesterol, or high blood pressure. In another study, he and epidemiologist Lisa Berkman of Yale University, reported that the risks of dying, if family and friends do not live nearby, are two to three times higher for men, and two to eight times higher for women.[10] The most frequent cause of death listed by the study was heart disease. As Abraham Lenzner, adjunct professor, clinical psychology, Dartmouth University, so aptly observed, "If you want to find out what is making a person sick, find out what's breaking his heart."[11]

Although the risk associated with living alone, without friends or relatives nearby, is greater for women, the mortality rate in the year that follows the death of a spouse is somewhat higher for men.[12] Reasons that have been suggested range from stereotypical gender roles, for example, meal preparation and housework, to emotional support. The good news is that a widower's risk of dying is only greater if he does not remarry. If he remarries, his chances of dying return to normal. (However, any correlation between late-life marriages and staying alive may be flawed, since men who remarry tend to be in better health and more energetic.[13])

A story of unlikely loneliness and isolation comes to mind. It was related to me by Leon Epstein, chairperson emeritus of Langley-Porter Neuropsychiatric Institute, University of California Medical School. The two children of an elderly woman who lived alone in one of San Franscisco's most affluent areas were worried about their mother. Their concern was so great that they decided to seek professional help, and were eventually referred to Epstein. "She seems different . . . hard to describe . . . just different," one of them said. At Epstein's suggestion, they brought their mother to his office. After introducing himself, Epstein asked the mother about the two young people with her. She said that she didn't know them, but that they were two of the "loveliest young people" she had met in a long time.

The story has a happy ending. The mother did not have Alzheimer's disease. Her condition was caused by malnutrition and was reversible. She lived alone, and although markets were nearby and she could afford to take a taxi or pay people to shop for her, she chose not to. Instead she stayed home and ate junk food. Two points: first, adequate income is important, but does not guarantee that an elderly person is doing well; and second, it can't be taken for granted that a child who lives nearby and visits on a regular basis will notice changes in a parent's condition. In Epstein's story, the mother and children had talked past one another for weeks, perhaps months, exchanging platitudes: "Isn't it a lovely day?" "The flowers are so beautiful." "You're looking good today."

Many of our elders survive for months or years on far less support than the woman in Epstein's story. Often the support is informal. At times it is improvised. A neighbor helps. A friend or church member comes by. I know of a situation in which the milk man not only put the milk in the refrigerator, but checked each day to see that his elderly customer was otherwise okay. What eventually happens, of course, is that informal support systems become unraveled. A neighbor moves. A friend dies or gets sick. Or the delivery company replaces the milk man. Still, the fact that such informal networks exist is in itself inspiring, and recalls the awe of Schopenhauer as he pondered our connectedness and the illusions that separate us from others.

No loss in late life is as complicated as the death of a spouse. In close and long-lived marriages, the mourning, and eventual healing, have been compared to tearing a piece of fabric in two and piecing it back together thread by thread.[14] Who turned off the alarm each morning? Who made the coffee? Who paid the bills? Who always remembered birthdays and special occasions?

There may even be, at times, a sense of the physical presence of the dead spouse, a deeply rooted instinctual quality that can be seen in the grief reactions of both human and nonhuman species, as in animal behaviorist Konrad Lorenz's description of bereavement in the greylag goose:

> The first response to the disappearance of the partner consists in the anxious attempt to find him again. The goose moves about restlessly by day and night, flying great distances and visiting places where the partner might be found, uttering all the time the penetrating trisyllabic call . . . The searching expeditions are extended further and further and quite often the searcher gets lost; or succumbs to an accident . . . [15]

There is a question among some social scientists as to whether the death of a spouse is as disabling for an elderly person as for a younger person.[16] Such comparisons miss the mark on two counts.

The first is that mourning, under any circumstances, at any age, and especially following the death of a spouse, is a highly individualized process and can't be quantified in a meaningful way. Speculations about how someone experiences grief cannot be isolated from the deeper existential question about how that individual chose to live his or her life.

The second reason is that death is *expected* in old age. We anticipate it. If we are even reasonably intelligent we prepare for it, and, consciously or unconsciously, rehearse it. Spousal bereavement, in late life, may seem less disabling simply because it occurs *on schedule*, so to speak, rather than *off schedule*. Sociologists refer to this kind of rehearsal as anticipatory socialization. Ecclesiastes described it more elegantly:

> To everything there is a season, and a time to every purpose under the heaven: a time to be born and a time to die . . .[17]

Lynch brings another dimension to our understanding of loneliness—the importance of the sound of the human voice; the mystery, as it were, of human dialogue. Human dialogue, he says, is the connection, or social synapse, that joins us together.

> What if we are far less distinct and separate than we have been led to believe? What if all our bodies are part of a much larger body— the communal body of mankind? Is human dialogue really a replacement for the umbilical cord we lose at birth, a tethered lifeline that continues to unite us all after birth? All of us drawing sustenance from one unseen common womb that we cannot feel because it engulfs us?[18]

Lynch's umbilical cord analogy recalls Stephen Daedelus's reflection in James Joyce's *Ulysses* as he looks at the midwife, "Mrs. Florence Mac Cabe, relict of the late Patk Mac Cabe, deeply lamented of Bride Street":

> One of her sisterhood lugged me squealing into life. . . . The cords of all link back, strand entwining cable of all flesh.[19]

The Healing Power of the Human Voice

Lynch goes further with his idea of speech as the membrane that unites us. It is, he suggests, not only the content of the dialogue, but the manner and tone of voice in which the dialogue is spoken.

An acquaintance comes to mind, a man in his early 60s whose loud, grating voice numbs everyone within earshot. I sometimes imagine birds shocked into stupor and falling from trees at the sound of his voice. One afternoon I heard him over the roar of a seaplane that was practicing landings and takeoffs on the lake behind our house. And he wasn't even shouting!

Until Lynch, my loyalties were one-sided. I had lined up with the environmentalists—unequivocally. However, the acquaintance I just mentioned warrants some concern. Each time he speaks, he drives up his blood pressure and accelerates his pulse, literally "red-lining" his vascular system. Fortunately all is not lost. Such people can improve their vascular health, and make the world more pleasant for the rest of us, simply by changing the way they speak. As with other forms of learned behavior, speech characteristics can be modified.

The elderly are especially vulnerable to speech/vascular interactions. Speaking elevates blood pressure in the elderly more than in younger people. The style of speaking itself, Lynch suggests, may contribute to inexplicable episodes of agitation—bursts of tempers—that seem to come out of the blue.[20] (A class in speech training for the elderly offers exciting possibilities.)

Equally important is teaching those who work with the elderly to enunciate rather than shout, to pitch their voices a little lower, and to adapt to the elderly person's speech rhythm. A constant fortissimo exhausts everyone within hearing range, and doesn't help any of us, old or young, to hear better.

The volume and quality of the human voice even affects animals. E. A. Bennet, an analytical psychologist, recalled a conversation with Carl G. Jung.[21] Jung told him that animals should be spoken to in whispers. This, Jung said, was told to him by a group of Franciscan monks in Switzerland whose ministry is healing animals—a practical, as well as humane, ministry in an area that specializes in farming.

It works. Titian, one of the four cats who share a house with my wife and me, was close to death from a kidney infection. He had been at an animal hospital in intensive care for several days and showed little improvement. Titian's wise and skilled veterinarian told me to take him home. He was neither eating nor taking fluids. If he was to recover, his doctor said, it would be in his home environment. After bringing him home, I followed Jung's advice by whispering encouraging words into his ear. His appetite for food and water was restored! There were other voices, too. As he slept in the basket on my desk, I played tapes of Mozart and Schubert continuously—not the sound of human dialogue, but, unquestionably, two of the voices of God.

Chapter 10

Fathers, Children, and Images of God

When Israel was a child I loved him, and I called my son out of Egypt.
> —Hosea

Fathers, provoke not your children to anger, lest they be discouraged.
> —St. Paul

We are the sons of our father, and we shall follow the print of his foot forever.
> —Thomas Wolfe, author of *Look Homeward Angel*

The fact that our parents, living or dead, affect us till the day we die is not a new idea. What they say and do to us from the time we are born, and perhaps even before, is with us always. More than other influences, their words and actions shape our personalities—according to Freud, by the time we are 5 to 7 years old.[1]

Even our health, as we move through midlife into late adulthood, appears to be influenced by our parents. This is underscored by a thirty-five-year followup of the Harvard Mastery of Stress Study, a highly regarded study carried out in the early 1950s. In that study, 126 healthy male undergraduates were subjects in two laboratory-administered stress tests, as well as a battery of psychological tests. Included in the psychological tests were two questions that called for open-ended narrative answers: "What kind of person is your mother?" and "What kind of person is your father?" The thirty-five-year followup correlated the responses with health status at midlife.

> Subjects who had illnesses such as coronary artery disease, hypertension, duodenal ulcer, and alcoholism at midlife had used significantly fewer positive words to describe their parents. . . . This effect was independent of subject's age, family history of illness, smoking behavior, marital history, and the death or divorce of the subject's parents. Furthermore, 95% of the subjects who used few positive words, and also rated their parents low in parental caring, had diseases diagnosed in midlife, whereas only 29 percent of subjects who used many positive words, and also rated their parents high in parental caring, had diseases diagnosed in midlife.[2]

This chapter, however, is not about both parents. It

is about the male parent only. Specifically it is about the importance of the male parent to the development of feelings of self-esteem and, in turn, to perceptions of God.

To begin, we are, without question, on firmer ground with father-son relationships than with father-daughter relationships. Sacred scripture, for example, is rife with father-son stories. In the New Testament, father-son stories range from the gentle beauty of Joseph and Jesus, to the eternal complexities of a father and his two sons in the parable of the prodigal son. There are no comparable father-daughter stories.

There is, of course, the story of the synagogue official whose daughter was restored to life by Jesus. But this is a miracle story, and only secondarily a story of a father-daughter relationship.

The obvious reasons, of course, center on the social history of the time, the patriarchy, and the then-inferior status of women. However, these reasons fall somewhat short of the mark. Many, if not most, of the followers of Jesus were women. The Gospel of St. Luke, for example, resonates to the feminine in both men and women. Why, then, the absence of father-daughter stories? I do not know. What it boils down to, I suggest, is a need for a sacred father-daughter story, a tale that will complement the "prodigal son" story, or its exquisite variant found in the Jewish tradition:

Kind Hearts

There was a king's son who went astray. The king sent a messenger telling the son to return to his father. The son said, "I cannot!" The king sent the messenger back. "Tell him," the king said, "to come as far as he can and I will come the rest of the way to him."[3]

After an extensive treatment of the mother-child relationship, Viorst writes of the importance of the male parent:

Our father presents an optional set of rhythms and responses for us to connect to. As a second home base, he makes it safer to roam. With him as an ally—a love—it is safer, too, to show that we're mad when we're mad at our mother. We can hate and not be abandoned, hate and still love. . . . And if we have no father, we will long for him.[4]

Viorst uses the term "father hunger." Father hunger, she says, is a "yearning for that other love" that "achievement and beauty, family and friends, even a cherished child" may never satisfy.[5]

Father hunger is sometimes expressed in unexpected ways, for example in dreams or synchronistic events. George, age 48, remembers his father as an angry, volatile man who died young. George was only 12. Years later, George met and married Martha. Martha had also lost her father, not to death, but to abandonment when she was 5 years old. After years of searching, she found him. Shortly afterward, George, thirty-six years from the date of his father's death, dreamed of a kind, gentle, elderly man with gray hair. In the dream the elderly man said that *he* was George's father. But instead of fear, he gave comfort and nurturance. Not his biological father, of course, but the ideal or archetypal father whose image George carried in his heart.

Here is another example. Carole's father is still living. She loves him deeply and he, in turn, loves her. Unfortunately, their love for one another was kept at arm's length by her father's alcohol addiction. Then the unexpected happened. As Jung says, "If you don't listen to life, life will turn around and hit you." And that is what happened to Carole's father. He fell down and narrowly escaped a crippling injury. During his rehabilitation he stopped drinking, and he and Carole have been able to realize the sacred gift of father-daughter love.

Finally, and sadly, is the story that a man named John told his analyst.[6] John was in his mid-30s. He described his father as a man who was always annoyed or irritated. About what, no one was certain. His father was a patient in a nursing home. It would be only a matter of months before he died, and John wanted to make one last attempt to bridge the distance between them. "Better a few months than none at all," he told his father.

"Do you want to know why we never got along?" his father asked.

"Yes."

"Well, I'll tell you. Do you remember the toy truck you broke because you couldn't get it to work? Or the GI Joe doll you tried to flush down the toilet? Do you remember how you lost the knife I gave you?" One story followed another until his emphysema forced him to stop. Then, with what breath remained, he said, "And that's why we could never get along."

John left the nursing home feeling that his burden had been lifted. "No child could have had a father relationship with that man," he thought. "Closure and love are out of the question."

Nemo tenetur ad inutile. Roughly translated, "One does not have a moral duty to do something that is useless." John's search for the father in his heart had begun. Hopefully, by the power and wonder of grace (or joss), John will cross paths with a male elder, a mentor who will become his spiritual father.

Among the elderly heart attack interviewees, comments about male parents correlated with high or low self-esteem.[7] These examples are from interviews with two women with low self-esteem scores:

> My father resented me. He used to threaten to slap me and make me work in the grocery store. He criticized everything, even the house [my husband] and I built on [a river] . . . He said the wood was no good.

My mother, I think, came from a religious family. But she married the wrong man. He didn't believe in church or anything else. . . . We never saw anything that pleased both of us. I was just waiting till I was old enough to get away from home.

Two men with low self-esteem scores remembered their fathers as having favored older brothers:

He called me Jack, but he called my older brother "Son" and that bothered me.

I have no qualms about my daddy except that he just didn't have time for me. [A long pause.] I have children. No matter what you do, you can't be fair to all of them. So I've forgotten about that part of it. But I can still see my daddy coming home with those two older boys. Both of them had watches. I couldn't figure out where mine was. Later on they got bicycles. I didn't get a bicycle. One time they both got wagons. I didn't get none. . . . I became resentful as I got older and older. [A long pause.] Then I was determined I would get the things I wanted.

In tandem with high or low self-esteem and memories of the male parent were contrasting perceptions of God; that is, perceptions of God as either benign and forgiving (high self-esteem interviewees) or punitive and vengeful (low self-esteem interviewees). These contrasting perceptions of God were especially intriguing, since several of the interviewees attended the same church, listened to the same sermons, went to the same Bible study classes, and probably regarded themselves as sharing similar religious views. Still, to some, God was benign and forgiving; to others, hostile and punitive.

Freud would not have been surprised. He argued that concepts of God derive from our experience, as infants and young children, with the authority of the male parent. The child, helpless and vulnerable, and the male parent, strong and invincible, mold the image the individual comes to recognize as God.[8] The Jesuit theologian William Johnston does not compare feelings about God to feelings about one's earthly father: he does, however, write of the importance of loving oneself in a relationship with a loving God.

> Fallen nature is full of mystery and contradiction. Alas, deep down in all of us is a tendency to hate ourselves and to destroy ourselves . . . Whatever the cause, some people have an acute sense of their own radical unlovableness. . . . this paralyzes them, making them reject love. Such people must learn to love themselves; and one way to do this is to accept the love of God and the love of people . . . [9]

Along similar lines, Dennis Linn and Matthew Linn, Jesuit priests, also wrote of self-perceptions and images of God.

> My image of God often tells me more about my image of myself than it does about God. To the degree that I love or hate myself, I will love and hate God, and vice versa. The real problem is not that we dislike God or our neighbor but that we don't like ourselves.[10]

Encouraging the interviewees to talk about religion was more difficult than I had imagined. Early in the interview, I asked a question about religion. Almost all of the responses were identical: "I go to church but I'm not a fanatic." There was obviously something more, so, toward the end of the interview, I returned to the question of religion. It was at that point that they described their personal beliefs in God. Their spiritual convictions were *always* consistent with the tenets of their churches, and were usually described in the context of experiences that grew out of their illnesses.

> A person trusts in God after he's been through this [a heart attack].

> A lot of people prayed for me . . . Might have deepened my convictions.

> Some people would say, "Why did God let this happen to me?" I feel, if anything, it brought me a little closer.

> I'm a Catholic . . . not a strong Catholic. Of course I do believe in prayer. One time I said [prayed to Jesus], "Your mother only suffered

until you were 33 years old and you were crucified. Now, why do I have to suffer longer?" Then I got a feeling that the Lord won't send you any more than you can take. I realized everything has a purpose.

Most of the high self-esteem interviewees described spiritual growth as a positive value that emerged from their illnesses. There were no similar comments among the interviewees with low self-esteem. An interviewee with low self-esteem said that he regretted not being a Christian, although he goes to church with his wife from time to time. I asked what he meant. He said that being a Christian required accepting the Bible, "every word of it," in a literal sense.

Another man with low self-esteem described days and nights of terror in the months following his bypass surgery. He said that he would lie in bed, afraid that he was going to die, and worry about sins he may have forgotten to confess. The terror became so intense that he asked the archbishop to come to his home and hear his confession:

> I think I was religious enough to where it hindered me. [Long pause.] I was so peculiar about confession. . . . he gave a general confession—absolution to dissolve all sins. I was concerned that I hadn't confessed all my sins. Before I was sick I thought I was in good shape. He [the archbishop] did that . . . wiped the slate clean.

I told him that must have been a wonderful experience and asked if it had helped. He said that it had helped, but not completely.

The importance of religion and church attendance to a patient's recovery following open-heart surgery is gaining widespread importance. A recent study concluded that the risk of death is three times greater for individuals who derive neither strength nor comfort from religion.

Those without any strength and comfort from religion had almost three times the risk of death as those with at least some strength and comfort. Similarly, not feeling deeply religious was associated with an increased risk of death. There was also a trend for infrequent attendance at religious services to be associated with an increased risk of death.[11]

An Afterthought

I am not a Freudian, although I have deep respect for many of Freud's insights. I obviously do not support his idea of God as an *illusion in the sense of a fiction*. I do, however, value his insight that suggests the male parent as the image of God that forms in the heart of a child. However, I would feel more compatible with his views had he identified the father as *one of the possible images*. There certainly may be others. For example, a friend recently told me that his grandmother is his God image. What becomes of that image, father or someone else, during the various stages of adulthood and late life remains a mystery—a mystery as unique to each of us as a thumbprint or DNA.

One thing more, a thought suggested to me by Richard Schmidt, an Episcopal priest, is that that projection of one's earthly god-image upon God is reciprocal rather than unilateral.[12] In other words, God, in turn, reflects something of God back upon one's feelings toward whoever happens to be his or her earthly god-image. This is consistent with a view of God as the archetypal creator, an ever-present, unending dynamic, who gives back in multiples all that is received.

Chapter 11

The Masks We Wear

I have formed a strong theory that there is no such thing as "turning into" a Nasty Old Man or an Old Witch. I believe that such people, and of course they are legion, were born nasty and witchlike, and that by the time they were about five years old they had hidden their rotten bitchiness and lived fairly decent lives until they no longer had to conform to rules of social behavior, and could revert to their original horrid natures.

—M. F. K. Fisher, author of
Sister Age

Jung chose the term *persona* to refer to the masks that each of us wear as we move from role to role—parent, worker, spouse, etc. The persona is identified with the masks of classic Greek drama. The masks were an integral part of the drama, and hence represent more than the token likenesses seen today at costume balls, worn as jewelry, or displayed by the thousands in the novelty shops of New Orleans during Mardi Gras. Although the masks have lost much of their power through years of trivialization, it is helpful to keep them in mind when we refer to the persona.

Each of us has a number of personae, probably four or five. Two are obvious: one for work, the other for home. Having more than three or four is difficult to handle. The persona, as Jungian analyst Harry Wilmer observed, "conceals our true nature and disguises both our shadow [those parts of ourselves that we wish were not there] and our finest ideals, yet it tries to approximate our ego ideal, so it is like putting on a face."[1]

I, for example, am a teacher, business person, husband, father, and companion to Skinner, an English springer spaniel. I have an ego-ideal that molds each persona in a way that is authentic to me, and hopefully appropriate to the situation at hand. It doesn't bother me if Skinner pulls me in directions I don't want to go, or drags me around in circles. However, a colleague who tries to make a fool of me is another matter.

I feel a deep love for my children and some of my students, but the love is quite different. So, too, is the persona I choose. In one instance, love is reflected through my parent persona; in the other, through my teacher persona.

The persona chosen may shift from role to role, but it is not phoniness. If the persona were only a mask, it would be seen through. It would be like living in a world of transparent and inauthentic people who behave like professional complaint handlers, tax agents, "warm and fuzzy" (yuk!) psychotherapists, or technicians who dazzle others with arcane terminology.

The danger of the persona is that it has the potential of taking over one's core personality. In such instances, discernment and common sense lose control, and the persona runs amok. The film actress Greta Garbo experienced such a takeover. After receiving bad reviews for one of her films, she retired and went into deep seclusion. She was only 36 years old. The reason she gave was that her legend was in peril. "My legend," she said, "is everything to me now. I would not sell it for life, happiness, or anyone . . . As a matter of fact I would even sacrifice my own life, so as not to jeopardize it."[2]

A persona out of control is a favorite dramatic theme. In the film *The Remains of the Day*, the manservant sacrifices love, authenticity, and even his humanness to fulfill his persona of chief of the household (butler). By the time he recognizes what has happened, it is too late.

More than 2,400 years ago, Euripides created a similar but less likable character in his play *The Trojan Women*. The play centers around the humiliation that was inflicted upon the women of a defeated enemy. Cassandra, describing the chief Greek herald, who, at the time, is reveling in his "lord and master" persona, says, "Why is it [that] heralds hold the name they do? All men unite in hating with one common hate the servants who attend kings and government."[3]

By late adulthood, we have had a lifetime of experience with the persona. Moreover, we have dealt with our personae in varying stages of transition, for example, from student to worker, wife or husband to widow or widower, worker to retiree, or homemaker to retirement-home resident. Still, the persona can take us by surprise, sometimes while we are interrelating with those closest to us. A moving example of an elderly-parent persona and an adult-child persona is told by the American dramatist S. N. Behrman in his autobiography. It is about the poet Siegfried Sassoon, a friend of Behrman's, and the dinner party at which Behrman first met Sassoon's mother:

> We were called into the dining room. Dinner was rather a trial . . . While I was talking, Siegfried's face grew darker and darker. I felt some sort of tension between him and his mother, the tension of great love but incomplete understanding.[4]

The feelings described by Behrman are familiar to anyone who works with the elderly and their children on a day-by-day basis. However, each parent-child relationship is, at heart, unique—a dyadic world unto itself. As the Russian novelist and philosopher Tolstoy wrote, "Happy families are all alike; each unhappy family is unhappy in its own way."[5]

From time to time painful revelations emerge. A man in his 50s told me about friends of his late mother who told him story after story about the light and whimsical side of her personality, a part of his mother he had never known. With sadness in his voice he said, "If only I had had *that* woman for my mother . . . I could have told *that* woman how much I loved her."

Equally sad is the story a woman told me about her late father-in-law, a man regarded by his family as bland and uninteresting. During family gatherings, he would retreat to his woodworking shop at the earliest possible moment. "Such a dull and boring man," my friend thought. After his death, the family decided to sell his tools and woodworking equipment. While cleaning his shop, they found several journals that he had kept. The family had no idea that the journals existed. The writings were a record of his dreams, reflections, and, at times, the anguish of that state of mind Thoreau described as "quiet desperation"[6]—so different from the man they remembered, that the journals might have been the work of a stranger.

Slightly less heartbreaking are the experiences of middle-aged children who find a previously undiscovered side of a parent only months, weeks, or days before that parent dies. Such experiences bring to mind the words of the American jurist Felix Frankfurter, who said that truth comes so seldom that we cannot fault it simply because it always seems to come too late.[7]

Here we must pause to make certain that the persona is kept in perspective. The feelings described by Behrman, Euripides, and Tolstoy are from the deepest levels of the human experience. But they are not personae. They are, however, reflected *through* a persona, as in the Greek drama when the voices of the actors were amplified through "larger than life" masks.

An analogy is to compare the total individual, in body, mind, and spirit, to a house. The persona is the house exterior, especially the doors and windows. Or, more accurately, the personae are a series of changing exteriors, windows, and doors; not the house itself, but an integral part of the house. The analogy is not altogether farfetched if we recall St. Teresa's spiritual classic, *Interior Castle*, in which the soul is envisioned "as if it were a castle . . . in which there are many rooms, just as in heaven there are many mansions."[8]

The persona in late adulthood is not to be dismissed. A striking example involved Robert W., an 83-year-old resident of a life-care retirement community in Sonoma, California. Robert and his 60-year-old wife moved to the retirement community from an expensive home in San Francisco. Mrs. W. did not want to move, but Robert insisted. Robert wanted to be certain that Mrs. W. would be well provided for after his death. It was important to him that she be left in handsome and expensive surroundings. However, Mrs. W. was angry from the day they moved into the retirement community. Within six weeks, shouting at Robert in a fit of pique, she keeled over and, two days later, died. Not more than a week or so after Mrs. W.'s death, Robert was stricken with a second tragedy. A son, in his 40s, was diagnosed with leukemia.

The other residents responded to Robert with compassion and, a few weeks later, elected him president of the Residents Association. It seemed a blessing at first. Then Robert's attorney persona surfaced. He was not only a gifted trial lawyer, but he specialized in one particular aspect of law—class-action suits. Robert's specialty was gathering together the dissident shareholders to sue the corporation. Soon the church-affiliated retirement community became analogous to a heartless corporation.

Residents who otherwise seemed relatively pleased with their lives began behaving like defrauded shareholders. Robert alleged that not only were funds being diverted to obscure missions in Third World countries, but earnings from a boutique that sold toiletry items were being siphoned off to buy furs and jewelry for wives of the management company. None of it made sense. But Robert contended wrongdoing with such power and conviction that almost all of the residents were swayed. It took a detailed and expensive audit, paid for by the residents, to assure them that nothing out of the ordinary was happening. Robert's rage, his skills as a trial lawyer, and his persona brimming with rectitude, created months of unhappiness for more than 150 elderly people, to say nothing of the board of directors and management personnel.

As a postlude, after the audit demonstrated that all was well, Robert continued as president of the Residents Association. His prestige did not drop one iota, even though his allegations were groundless, unnecessary, worrisome, and very expensive.

To the relief of many, Robert decided to return to a part-time law practice. He handled the estates of several residents and was a volunteer advisor to many charitable and civic organizations.

During the ordeal of the audit, Robert and I became friends. I liked him in spite of what was happening. I enjoyed his stories of legal battles won against overwhelming odds. He lived to be 90 years old and died in the nursing-home section of the retirement community. His only request to me during the months he was in the nursing home was that a case of his favorite Scotch whisky be kept where he could see it from his bed. Needless to say, I complied.

Late adulthood is a last call for authenticity, a last chance to deal with pretense. It is also a time when masks, pretense, and personae may be more complicated than ever, as in the experience told to me by a retiree in his 70s:

At a party, when someone asks me about myself, especially if they ask how I'm enjoying retirement, I can never give an appropriate or even sensible answer. Instead of saying, "It's fine," or something like that, I give an answer that sounds like a Who's Who listing. My answer describes what I once was, but not what I am now. I need an "emeritus" status, real estate broker emeritus, for example. As dumb as it sounds, I need something more than simply "retiree." Only once have I been able to describe myself as what I am: a decent human being. Even then I felt awkward for the rest of the evening. I felt as though I had been flippant and ill-mannered.

With deference to my friend's plight, I am not certain that an emeritus persona would do more good than harm. Perhaps in the long run it would thwart the personal growth that Jung regarded as characteristic of the second half of adulthood.

Jung says that the tasks and goals of the first half of adulthood are quite different than those that occur after reaching midlife. In "life's morning," using Jung's term, goals and concerns are externally directed—establishing a career, marrying, rearing children, defining one's place in society, etc. At midlife, the beginning of "life's afternoon," the emphasis gradually shifts from external to internal concerns, and focuses on intrapsychic growth and matters of spirit, wholeness, and soul:

But we cannot live the afternoon of life

according to the programme of life's morning; for what was great in the morning will be little at evening, and what in the morning was true, will at evening have become a lie.[9]

On a positive note, and in line with Jung's views, the retiree-persona dilemma is seen less frequently now than, say, fifteen or twenty years ago. Sometimes it isn't seen at all. Its absence is refreshing.

I was made aware of its absence a few months ago during an Elderhostel (a program of one-week college courses for people aged 60 and over).[10] It was Friday afternoon and the week of classes was over. As I was saying goodbye to one of the students, a man in his late 60s, he said, "What I liked best about this week was that not once did I hear anybody talk about what they *used to do* or what they *used to be*." I thought of my 70-year-old friend. In this setting, would he have found it necessary to revive his midlife persona? To bring it out of storage for all to see? Or, instead, simply and quietly, would he have relished the present, the here and now, the moment God had given.

Chapter 12

Wise Old Fools

> If you want your children to be brilliant, tell them fairy tales. If you want them to be very brilliant, tell them even more fairy tales.
>
> —attributed to the physicist Albert Einstein[1]

This chapter is about the wisdom of foolishness. It is based on a fairy tale about an old man who lost a fortune twice before regaining it in an unexpected way.

But first, a word about fairy tales. Fairy tales are good stories with happy endings. People have been entertained by them for centuries. No one ever said that they really happened. Still, their truths, although not literal or factual, are often profound.

Most fairy tales about older people do not have a single sprightly creature in them. Unlike tales about young people, relatively few fairy tales about older people include kings, queens, or royalty. Most of them are about ordinary people in extraordinary circumstances. The stories tell about how they got into such situations and managed to get out again.

Fairy tales are meant to entertain. But they are also "teaching stories"—they teach values and lessons that are eternally fresh. This is due in part to the need of fairy tales to be *told* rather than *read*. Each person who tells the story brings something new to it. Over time, that which is essential and vital remains. That which no longer has a purpose is deleted, modified, or slowly fades away.

Allan Chinen[2], a Jungian analyst and a member of the clinical faculty of the University of California Medical School in San Francisco, is probably the foremost scholar of fairy tales about elderly people. His extensive and meticulous research is based on an analysis of more than four thousand fairy tales, of which about two percent have an older person as protagonist.

Chinen uses the term "elder tales" rather than "fairy tales." I use the terms interchangeably, even though there are substantive differences in the psychological structure of fairy tales about older persons as opposed to younger persons. Fairy tales about younger persons deal with the tasks of growing up. Fairy tales about older persons deal with the tasks of growing inward, both psychologically and spiritually. In tales about young people, we learn about physical dangers and the merits of acquiring what is one's due, against all odds. In fairy tales about older persons we learn about tending to the soul. Fairy tales about young people move outward. Those about older persons move inward.

Fairy tales and dreams have much in common. Each is part of the language of the unconscious, rich with symbolism, and concerned with matters of soul more than intellect. Another similarity is that a single fairy tale, like a single dream, may not make much sense. But if put side by side with other tales, recurrent themes emerge that yield deeper and richer insights. Finally, both fairy tales and dreams are set in the *liminal*. By liminal, I refer to a particular space or period of time in a ritual, or transitional, process; specifically, that particular space or period of time between separation (an ending) and reincorporation (a new beginning):

Separation —> Liminality —> Reincorporation

or:

Ending —> Neutral Zone —> New Beginning

Thus, a liminal state is an in-between or fallow state.[3] For that reason, fairy tales usually take place on the edge of the forest, the edge of the sea, or next to a river: in other words, the symbolic edge of the unconscious.

Many of our elders exist in a state of perpetual liminality. This is especially so in situations where elderly people are forced to survive on inadequate incomes, eating one meal a day, sometimes having to choose between eating or paying their electric bill. Sadly, there is little hope of things getting better. This is what anthropologist Maria Vesperi meant when she described the low-income elderly in St. Petersburg, Florida, as being stranded in the liminal, with death as their only exit.[4]

In fairy tales about old people, the protagonists are almost always in a liminal state. But through a remarkable, often outrageous, sequence of events, the liminal becomes not only bearable, but transcendent. The story I have chosen is such a story. It is from Italy and is about an old man who finds deliverance in his foolishness. It is freely adapted from Chinen's book. (Parts of this tale may seem sexist to the modern reader, but it is representative of its time, and as a fairy tale it would not work otherwise.)

The Shining Fish[5]

Once upon a time, an old man and his wife lived in a house that overlooked the sea. Their children had all died, and they were poor and alone. The old man eked out a living by gathering wood in a nearby forest and selling it in the village. One day, while gathering wood, he met a wise man with a long gray beard. "I know all about your troubles," the stranger said, "and I want to help."

He gave the old man a small leather bag. When the old man opened it, he almost fainted. It was full of gold! By the time he came to his senses, the stranger was gone. The old man threw away his wood and rushed home. But along the way he began to think: "If I tell my wife about this money, she will waste it all." So when he arrived home, he said nothing. Instead he hid the money in a pile of manure.

The next morning, the old man awakened to the aroma of breakfast. "Where did you find the money for breakfast?" he asked his wife. "You did not bring home any wood to sell," she said, "so I sold the manure." The old man shrieked. Then he jumped up and ran out of the house, into the forest.

He went back to work, chopping wood and muttering and cursing to himself. Then the stranger with the long beard appeared again. He laughed and said to the old man, "I know what you did with the money, but I still want to help." So he gave the old man another purse filled with gold. The old man rushed home, but along the way he once again

Kind Hearts

thought: "If I tell my wife, she will squander this fortune." This time he hid the gold in a pile of rags. The next morning he awakened to find that his wife was again cooking a hearty breakfast. "You did not bring back any firewood," she explained, "so I sold the rags."

The old man ran into the forest, beside himself with anger. Again he met the stranger with the long beard. The stranger smiled sadly and said, "My friend, some people are not destined to be rich, and it seems that you are one of them. But I still want to help." He gave the old man a large bag. Instead of gold, the bag contained twenty-four frogs. "Take the frogs and sell them in the village. Then use the money to buy the largest fish you can find—not dried fish, shellfish, sausages, cakes, or bread—the largest fish!" With that, the stranger vanished.

The old man hurried to the village and sold the frogs. He saw many wonderful things that he wanted to buy, but he followed the stranger's advice and bought the largest fish he could find. He returned home late in the evening. He was too tired to clean the fish, so he hung it outside the house and went to bed.

That night it stormed. The old man and his wife could hear the waves crashing against the rocks below their house. Then, in the middle of the night, they were awakened by someone pounding on the door. The old man opened the door and found a group of young fishermen standing outside. "Thank you for saving our lives!" they said.

"What do you mean?" the old man asked. The fishermen explained: they were caught at sea by the storm and did not know which way to row, until they saw a light shining from the old couple's house. "A light?" asked the old man.

"Yes," they said, pointing to the fish, which was hanging from the rafters and shining with such brightness that it could be seen for miles. "Because you have saved our lives," the captain of the fishing boat said, "you and your wife will never be without food. For as long as you live, we will share our catch with you."

Every night, from that time on, the old man hung a shining fish outside the house to

guide the young fishermen home. The fishermen, in turn, shared their catch with him and
his wife! And so the old couple lived in comfort and honor the rest of their days.

Chinen's interpretation is both rich and insightful. I
will touch upon a few of his points:
The setting includes both the edge of the forest and
the edge of the sea—the *liminal* in every sense of the
word. That is where the old man and his wife live. They
have endured both poverty and loss. Not only have they
struggled to make ends meet, but they have suffered
losses from which grief is unremitting: the deaths of
their children.

The benefactor, however, comes from *deep* in the
woods—the *unconscious.* In other words, a part of the
unconscious is trying to break into consciousness. If
successful, it will be the old couple's deliverance.

The symbolism of the story moves from "gold" to
"frogs" to a "large and luminous fish." Gold is the color
of the sun and represents human consciousness. In this
story, it is a gift that is given and lost twice and, therefore, must be important. Frogs symbolize the transformative. During Easter season, tadpoles turn into frogs
and are symbolic of the Resurrection. The symbolism
then moves from the transformative to wholeness in the
form of a fish, the symbol of Jesus Christ.

Thus, the story moves from:

gold —>	frog —>	fish
(human	(transformation/	(Jesus Christ/
consciousness)	resurrection)	self/wholeness)

Chinen also emphasizes the old man's weakness: money. This is understandable, since he's always been without it. Money overwhelms him. It seduces him. Worse, it tricks him into mistaking wiliness for intelligence. He hides the gold from his wife, for selfish reasons, and, of course, loses it twice. Finally, with the third try, he reaches, or is kicked into, a new level of consciousness. Instead of trying to outsmart others, he follows the instructions of his benefactor to the letter. The benefactor with the long gray beard may symbolize God or the image of God carried in our hearts.

Another theme suggested by Chinen is generativity, that is, fostering the growth and development of the next generation. By his actions, the old man unwittingly fosters the growth and well-being of others younger than himself—the fishermen. The old man saved their lives and, without knowing it, affirmed his connectedness to the universe.

Each interpretation is brilliantly developed by Chinen. I agree without reservation. However, no single interpretation is the only interpretation. Fairy tales have a mercurial quality—they are transformative by nature, and continue to change according to time and circumstance. In this respect, too, fairy tales are similar to dreams. As the meaning of a dream emerges from the dreamer, so does the meaning or particular interpretation of the fairy tale emerge from the storyteller. Hence there are always differences in interpretation.

Another interpretation is that, although the gold would have made the old man wealthy, it may not have made him happy. The story tells us that he had problems with money. Otherwise he would not have hidden the money from his wife. Like so many lottery or sweepstake winners, the wealth probably would have brought problems and challenges that the old man and his wife were not prepared to deal with. As the wise man said, the old man was not meant to be rich. Still, he is a good person and deserves a reward. As it turns out, the reward is sustenance rather than wealth. Not riches in the form of gold, but an annuity, so to speak, in the form of fish.

Coming to terms with one's lot is a task of the second half of life. It is the stage of life when we modify or redefine the limits of our dreams and ambitions. And what better symbol of dreams and ambition than gold? If we are wise, we let go of the gold. If not, like the old man, we lose it.

James F. T. Bugental,[6] an existential psychotherapist, refers to such insights as coming to terms with the "nevers": "I'm never going to be president of the company

. . . never going to be a great pianist . . . never going to play tennis like Arthur Ashe. The "nevers" is consistent with William James's paradigm of ideal self (or pretense) gradually giving way to actual self (or reality). Such insights, James observed, always come as a "blessed relief."[7]

Giving way to the inevitable is not all loss. Sometimes there is enormous gain, as in the Japanese story "The Stonecutter."[8]

Once upon a time there was an old stonecutter who was very unhappy about his lot in life. Day after day he cursed his fate. One day, in anguish, he looked to the heavens and said, "Ruler of the Universe, I can tolerate my misery no longer. Make me rich and powerful." And his wish was granted.

Then one day, perspiring in the heat of the sun, he said, "Ruler of the Universe, the sun is more powerful than I am. Make me into the sun." And his wish was granted. Then one day his brightness was obscured by a cloud. He said, "Ruler of the Universe, that cloud is more powerful than the sun. Make me into a cloud." And his wish was granted. Then one day he drifted into a mountain peak. The mountain was oblivious to him and that made him angry. "Ruler of the Universe," he said, "that mountain is more powerful than a cloud. Make me into a mountain." And his wish was granted.

He enjoyed being a mountain until one day he felt pain in his feet. He looked down and saw a stonecutter chopping away at the base of the mountain. "Master of the Universe," he said, "that stonecutter is more powerful than I. Make me into a stonecutter." And his wish was granted. Once again he was a stonecutter. But now he was content with himself.

The stonecutter moves, from envy and craving for what he is not, to acceptance and affirmation of what he truly is. His journey brought him back to where he began. But along the way he gave up his pretensions. He returned "to his old job with a new, wider, perspective—a glimpse of the larger picture and an understanding of his small place within a greater drama."[9]

Another interpretation is that the two men in the first story are composite figures: the ordinary, perhaps foolish, old man (the beneficiary), and the deity or wise man (the benefactor). Each without the other is lacking and incomplete. Together they are whole.

No doubt the impoverished old man needs the wisdom of the wise man. He has much inner work to do. Because of his bungling, the gold was lost, not once, but twice. But if he hadn't lost his gold, he wouldn't have bought the fish, and the young fishermen would have drowned. Further, if the ordeal of losing a fortune two days in a row hadn't exhausted him, he more than likely would have had the energy to clean and eat the fish. Instead he hung it on the rafters (contemptuously, perhaps), and went to bed. Like the Christian concept of grace, the magic returned unexpectedly and without effort.

By the same token, the wise man is also incomplete. He may be "all-knowing," but he is stifling. He needs something more. He needs the humanness and humility of the old wood-gatherer and, at least, a modicum of foolishness. A touch of foolishness may be the gift to the wise man from his otherwise impoverished counterpart.

Jung said that we too frequently treat the old fool with disdain.[10] We forget that when we look back on our lives, what really counted and made the difference often came not from wisdom, planning, or foresight, but from life's unexpected detours. Some real-life examples:

> Aniela Jaffe, who was Jung's assistant in his last years, described her marriage at a young age as foolishness. Both she and her husband were too young for the marriage to succeed.

Kind Hearts

But as a result of her marriage, she obtained a Swiss passport and eventually traveled to study with Jung.

Joseph Campbell, after studying in France for years, returned to Columbia University to complete his dissertation. However, the narrowness of the structure of a dissertation discouraged him. With only a year remaining to complete his doctorate, he sought a broader vision. Years later he finished writing his classic *The Hero with a Thousand Faces* and began his meteoric career as a writer and teacher.

As a young man, journalist Bill Moyers wanted to become a Baptist minister. Somewhere along the way he made a detour, and instead became one of the premier interviewers of our day.

Each person took a detour that, at the time, must have seemed foolish, if not catastrophic. But in the long run each detour turned out well. Jean Houston has an exercise in which she asks each participant taking her workshop to name his or her greatest blunder. I use the same exercise in my classes on life transitions. Since most of my students are at midlife and have had a number of life experiences, the results are often amazing. More frequently than imagined, the important things that happened to them began with a detour.

What seems foolish in our elders is often not foolishness at all. It is simply doing what is acceptable if you are young, but unacceptable if you are old. My favorite TV series brings this point home with humor and panache. The show is *Waiting for God*, produced in the United Kingdom and aired on public television. In each sequence, Tom and Diana, two elderly residents of a retirement home, are at odds with the home's administrator. The administrator wants to maintain an atmosphere of decorum and propriety—a proper home for English ladies and gentlemen. But Tom, Diana, and the other residents will not let that happen. They will not succumb to the stereotype, which leads to story lines full of romance, sex, and political intrigue, not to mention confrontations with issues like death, insensitive health-care providers, and deadly-dull children.

To the home's administrator, and Tom's son and daughter-in-law, Tom and Diana appear dotty and foolish. Nonetheless, in each confrontation Tom and Diana win, and the administrator, dubbed the "Idiot" Baines, is thwarted. Tom and Diana may be weaker and more vulnerable than their adversaries, but they are wiser, smarter, and more experienced. Tom and Diana refuse to yield to conventional mores. Appearing foolish in the eyes of others does not affect them in the least.

Harry Wilmer[11] quotes Jung as saying that the wise old fool is our best teacher, and that wisdom is found more often in foolishness than in cleverness. There is, however, a barb. Paraphrasing Jung, Wilmer says that although foolishness itself requires no art, there is, nonetheless, an art to be found and appreciated. And that art—perhaps the crowning task of a life fully lived—is the art of extracting wisdom out of foolishness.

Epilogue

Two milestone events happened to me while I was working on this book: I had open-heart surgery (aortic valve replacement) and I turned 65. Because of my work with heart attack survivors, the experiences of life after heart surgery came as no surprise. As to turning 65, there were surprises, but, all in all, not as many as when I turned 60, which was my father's age at the time of his death.

Heart surgery has meant more to me than simply staying alive. It was an experience during which I had to give up control of much of what happened to me. I prepared myself psychologically and spiritually. I also selected the Schubert and Mozart tapes that I would play continuously during my stay in the hospital. But that was it. The surgery was performed by a team of people who, until the morning of surgery, were strangers to me. I had, of course, met the surgeon, but had not talked with him more than two or three times. The cardiologists who diagnosed the valve disease, and eventually recommended surgery, are known to me professionally. It would have been comforting to have had a good friend as a doctor or member of the hospital staff. But I didn't. I simply trusted, and the results could not have been better.

Heart surgery also affirmed the importance of my family. Carol, my wife, was with me day and night. Both my daughter, Gloria, and son, Michael, came from San Francisco to Mobile to be with me—Gloria before and during my hospitalization, and Michael during my first two weeks at home. I cherish the blessing expressed by their love.

Being fully alive and aware of the joys of the five senses is another gift. The words of the poet W. H. Auden comes to mind:

> Be happy, precious five,
> So long as I'm alive
> Nor try to ask me what
> You should be happy for
> Think, if it helps, of love
> Or alcohol or gold
> But do as you are told.[1]

Knowing that my heart beats, and knowing that I am alive with my precious five senses intact, because the aortic valve I was born with has been replaced by a porcine (pig) valve, is both humbling and exhilarating. It links two seemingly incongruent emotions: On the one hand, I am awed by the accomplishments of science; on the other, I am kept from ego-inflation by the knowledge that I was saved by a pig's aortic valve.

Turning 65 meant more to me than I thought it would. But first, an aside: Age 65 has no psychological, social, or physiological meaning. It is an age selected in the nineteenth century by Otto von Bismarck, Germany's Iron Chancellor, as the age when old-age pensions would begin. In the 1930s our legislators needed a qualifying age for Social Security, and Bismark's choice, age 65, was as good as any. Sensible or not, however, age 65 is an age of initiation, ritualized by such things as going to the Social Security office, receiving a Medicare card, and, if you are male, being on the mailing list of almost every impotence clinic in America.

Turning 65 gave me membership in a group that I have spent the better part of my adult years studying. I am no longer an outsider looking in. Now, instead, I am one of those people termed senior citizens, who live in the land of the young—a Struldbrugg, as Jonathan Swift called them in *Gulliver's Travels*. Or, in today's jargon, I'm a "geezer." However, I do not feel any different.

An advantage of being 65 is that now I can talk about aging from the point of view of an insider. For certain, there is a difference between the "young old" and the "old old"—as much as an entire generation. Still, the bottom line is that age 65 is a ritual age. I have crossed it and, so far, all is well.

Heart surgery and turning 65 have intensified my feelings of thankfulness. I have made it a practice to give thanks as a daily meditation. The results are always uplifting, and it is easy to do. I simply give thanks for blessings, both present and past: for example, parents, spouse, friends who helped along the way (I name them), children, animals (I name them, too), sunny days, cloudy days (good for the soul), rainy days, fine restaurants, music, books, art, mechanical devices that work, and, most of all, unexpected blessings, as in the poem by the distinguished New England poet Robert Frost:

> The way a crow
> Shook down on me
> The dust of snow
> From a hemlock tree
> Has given my heart
> A change of mood
> And saved some part
> Of a day I had rued.[2]

Naomi Remen uses a similar exercise in her work with cancer patients. The act of thanksgiving, she says, is central to the healing process: sometimes patients spend hours giving thanks for things that happened years before, but were never acknowledged.[3]

Brother David Steindl-Rast, a Benedictine monk, says that thankfulness is prayer, and prayer, in turn, is thankfulness. It is anticipatory thankfulness, as in saying "Please" when we ask for something. Brother David quotes a mystic who resonated to the word of God: "You would not search for Me if you had not already found Me."[4]

Try the exercise. If you do not believe in prayer, then a litany of thankfulness, at least, will relax you and make you feel better. If you do believe in prayer, a litany of thankfulness will not only relax you and make you feel better, but at some point, the two, thankfulness and prayer, will cease being separate, and become one.

Appendix

Research Methodology: Elderly Heart Attack Survivors

> No test instrument has been devised that admits reliable information about the meaning of an event to a person.
>
> —Herbert Weiner

The purpose of the study was to identify those psychosocial qualities that protect an individual's self-esteem in the event of a life-threatening illness. The methodology[1] consisted of developing hypotheses; selecting a specific type of life-threatening illness; finding volunteer subjects who had experienced the onset of that illness during late adulthood; administering two questionnaires to a group of subjects and, identifying two subgroups, namely individuals with *high* and *low* self-esteem; interviewing in depth those persons who scored high and those who scored low on both questionnaires; and analyzing the data.

The hypotheses were suggested by a combination of

classic and contemporary theories on the concept of self, by literature that deals with life-threatening illnesses in late adulthood, by prevalent gerontological self-esteem theories, and by an exhaustive search of research literature on the self, as referenced in the *Index Medicus* during a twenty-four-year period from 1960 to 1984.

The reason for choosing subjects who had experienced a heart attack, rather than some other type of life-threatening illness, was that the precipitating mechanisms of a coronary occur in a manner that is reasonably similar in adults of all ages. For this reason, a heart attack is more indicative than other long-term illnesses in delineating age-related differences.

Subjects were selected based upon the following criteria:

- a first heart attack was experienced after the age of 60;

- the heart attack occurred more than a year prior to the study;

- there were no confounding influences upon self-esteem during the past year (for example, onset of other life-threatening illnesses, death of a spouse, divorce or marital separation, death or life-threatening illness of children or grandchildren);

- absence of economic hardship;

- non-institutionalization (that is, subjects were community-dwelling and were not patients in

Kind Hearts

a hospital or nursing home).

The subjects completed two self-esteem question-naires: Coppersmith's "Self-Esteem Inventory" and Rosenberg's "Self-Esteem Scale."[2] The questionnaires identified two subgroups: high scorers and low scorers. To qualify as an interviewee, the subject had to score either high or low on both questionnaires. Subjects who scored high on one questionnaire and low on the other were not interviewed.

The questionnaires were scored. Persons with the six highest scores on both questionnaires, and persons with the six lowest scores on both questionnaires, were interviewed in depth, using a semi-structured interview format.

The choice of an in-depth interview instrument—that is, a qualitative rather than quantitative approach—is in line with Bugental's[3] comments pertaining to the inability of traditional psychological research methods to deal with the nonmeasurable aspects of human beings. Interviewing is especially appropriate in dealing with topics that have deep personal meanings, a criterion that seems particularly apt in searching for the factors that protect an elderly individual from the erosion of self-esteem following a heart attack.

The interviews were taped and notes were taken to record gestures or actions that seemed meaningful. The tapes were transcribed by hand to facilitate searching for thematic content. This enabled an almost microscopic concentration on each interview item: the statement itself, the sound of the voice, hesitations, pauses, etc. An established technique of thematic analysis of content was used.[4] Researcher expectations were controlled by studying each transcript as a whole, and then by abstracting and classifying interviewee statements according to their relevance to particular hypotheses.

There were acknowledged limitations:

- The small number of subjects, all of whom are white and financially secure, precluded conclusions that can be generalized. Nor did it take into account ethnic or economic differences that may affect self-esteem.

- The disadvantages of a self-selected sample; that is, persons who are willing to talk about feelings of self-worth following a coronary may have higher feelings of self-esteem, and healthier personality functioning, than would be found in a random selection.

- Although each of the subjects had experienced a heart attack, no information was available regarding the degree of severity of their illnesses, which is an important correlate to psychological health.[5] However, information on subsequent cardiac illness, which is also a contributing factor, was available from a Basic Information Sheet and interview content.

Kind Hearts

Chapter Notes

Chapter 1

1. The demographics are from a number of sources: Hayflick, *How and Why We Age*, p. 70; McLean, "The Graying of America," pp. 22–31; Skinner & Vaughan, *Enjoy Old Age*. The AARP reference is from Dychtwald & Flower, *Age Wave: The Challenge and Opportunity of an Aging America*, p. 55.

2. Butler, *Why Survive? Being Old in America*.

3. Atchley, *Social Forces and Aging* (6th ed.), p. 280. Probably the most frequently used text in the field of social gerontology.

4. Clark & Anderson, *Culture and Aging: An Anthropological Study of Older Americans*.

5. "Oregon to fund assisted suicide for poor." *Housing for the Elderly Report*.

6. *The Jerusalem Bible*, Dn. 13.

7. Ibid., Dt. 5:16.

8. *Holy Bible* (King James Version), Ps. 71:9.

9. *The Jerusalem Bible*, Qo. 12:1–2; 4–5

10. Shakespeare, *Hamlet*, II, ii, 223; 406

11. Shakespeare, *King Lear*, II, iv, 145–149. A comprehensive treatment of old age in literature is found in de Beauvoir, *The Coming of Age*, Ch. 5–8.

12. Grotjahn, in Blythe, *The View in Winter: Reflections of Old Age*, p. 36.

13. Swift, *Gulliver's Travels*, III, Ch. 10.

14. Melamed, *Mirror, Mirror: The Terror of Not Being Young*, p. 9.

15. de Beauvoir, *The Coming of Age*, p. 299.

16. Belsky, *The Psychology of Aging: Theory, Research & Interventions* (2nd ed.), pp. 51–52.

17. In addition to Atchley, op. cit., the reader is directed to Palmore (Ed.), *Normal Aging: Reports from the Duke Longitudinal*

Study, Vols. I & II.

18. Adapted from a Sufi story told by Idries Shah.

19. Viorst, *Necessary Losses*, pp. 339–340.

20. Frush, *Self-Esteem in Older Persons Following a Heart Attack: An Exploration of Contributing Factors*.

21. Jung, *Memories, Dreams, Reflections*, p. 297.

22. Yeats, *Collected Poems*, p. 92.

Chapter 2

1. Rosenberg, *Society and the Adolescent Self-Image*, p. 31.

2. McDougall, *The Energies of Men* (3rd ed.), p. 234.

3. Allport, *Personality: A Psychological Interpretation*, p. 171.

4. Becker, *The Denial of Death*, p. 6.

5. Levin, "Age Stereotyping: College Student Evaluations," pp. 89–93.

6. McLean, op. cit., p. 23. The Rowe quote originally appeared in *Newsweek*.

7. Confusing self-esteem and self-concept is an inherent flaw in the arguments of both proponents and opponents of state-funded self-esteem task forces, for example, in responses to the California Task Force to Promote Self-Esteem and Personal Social Responsibility.

8. Chopra, *Creating Health*, p. 106.

9. Cortis, *Heart and Soul*, p. 88.

10. James, *The Principles of Psychology*, p. 200.

11. Taylor, "Adjustment to Threatening Events: A Theory of Cognitive Adaptation." Also, Neugarten, "Personality and Aging," pp. 626–649.

12. Frush, op. cit.

13. Jaffe, *Healing From Within*, p. 125.

14. Remen, "The Eye of an Eagle, the Heart of a Lion, the Hand of a Woman."

15. James, op. cit., p. 188 ff.

16. George, "Financial Security in Later Life: The Subjective Side."

17. James, op. cit., p. 200.

18. From a promotional video hosted by Kaye Stevens, *Life in Prime Time.*

19. Cooley, *Human Nature and the Social Order,* p. 246.

20. Winkelvoss & Powell, *Continuing-Care Retirement Communities: An Empirical, Financial, and Legal Analysis,* p. 13.

21. Erikson, "Generativity and Ego Integrity," pp. 85–87.

22. Miller, *Death of a Salesman.* Requiem.

23. Jung, "The Stages of Life," p. 19.

24. Auden, in Baraseh, *The Healing Path,* p. 390.

25. Kopp, *If You Meet the Buddha on the Road, Kill Him!,* p. 4.

Chapter 3

1. Frush, op. cit., pp. 83–86.

2. Wilhelm & Baynes (Trans.) *I'Ching.*

3. Ibid. Carl G. Jung, "Forward," XXXIX.

4. Bolin, *The Tao of Psychology.*

5. May, *The Cry for Myth.* p. 118. An excellent treatment of the psychology of Hermes can be found in Stein, *In Midlife: A Jungian Perspective.*

6. Adapted freely from Herodotus's *The History.*

7. Herodotus, *The History,* p. 98.

8. Seligman, *Learned Optimism.*

9. Ibid., pp. 15–16.

10. Ibid., p. 44.

Chapter 4

1. Pascal, *Pensees,* p. 222.

2. Keen & Moyers, *Your Mythic Journey.* Also, Keen, *Telling Your Story.*

3. Ibid.

4. In Feinstein & Krippner, *Personal Mythology,* pp. 18–21.

5. Keen & Moyers, op. cit.

6. An exercise suggested by Carol Frush.

7. Jung, *Memories, Dreams, Reflections,* p. 3.

8. Kopp, op. cit., p. 21.

9. A reflection suggested by Hazel Woodward.

10. de Beauvoir, op. cit., p. 288.

11. Ibid, p. 303.

12. Ibid, p. 298.

13. Butterfield, "Of Lineage and Love," p. 12.

14. Viorst, op. cit., pp. 339–340.

15. Told to me by Leon Epstein.

16. Lewis, "For Whom the Job Bell Doesn't Toll."

17. Medoff and others are cited in "Middle-aged Men Risk Layoffs." In another article, "Job Bias Complaints Swamp Investigators," it is suggested that old-age bias complaints are riding on the coattails of burgeoning sex, disability, and race bias complaints, which have accelerated in numbers since the American Disabilities Act, 1990. Both articles appeared in the *Mobile Register*.

18. Bly (Trans.), *The Kabir Book: Forty-four of the Ecstatic Poems of Kabir*, p. 2.

19. Seligman, op. cit., p. 75.

20. Yalom, *Love's Executioner*, p. 217.

Chapter 5

1. Erikson, Erikson & Kivnick, *Vital Involvement in Old Age*, 1986.

2. Ibid, p. 71.

3. Viorst, op. cit., p. 261.

4. Percy, *Lanterns on the Levee*, p. 347.

5. *Heart Letter*, p.7.

6. *The Jerusalem Bible*, Mt. 5:38–42.

7. Ibid, Mt. 10:23.

8. Linn & Linn, *Healing Life's Hurts: Healing Memories Through the Five Stages of Forgiveness*.

9. *The Book of Common Prayer*, Ps. 69:14–16; 30.

10. Pope John Paul II, "A Message to the Elderly."

Chapter 6

1. De Tocqueville, *Democracy in America*, Vol. II, p. 106.

2. Emerson, *Self-Reliance.*

3. A study performed in the early 1970s by Cory, Canapary, and Galanis for Casa Dorinda, a retirement community located in Montecito, California.

4. O'Bryant, "Older Widows and Independent Life Styles," pp. 41–51.

5. As in Cooley, op. cit., p. 246.

6. Butterfield, op. cit., pp. 14–15.

7. Erikson, *Childhood and Society* (rev. ed.). See also Erikson, "Generativity and Ego Integrity," pp. 85–87. Erikson divided the life span into eight stages. Each stage is highlighted by, and named after, a specific developmental task, the completion of which always involves a turning point or psychosocial crisis. Briefly, the crises, and approximate ages at which they occur, are: (1) Basic Trust versus Basic Mistrust (first year of life); (2) Autonomy versus Shame and Doubt (second year); (3) Initiative versus Guilt (third to fifth years); (4) Industry versus Inferiority (between seventh and eleventh years); (5) Identity versus Identity Confusion (puberty to about age 20); (6) Intimacy versus Isolation (early adulthood); (7) Generativity versus Stagnation (adulthood, mid-life); (8) Integrity versus Despair (late adulthood and old age). The boundaries of the eight psychosocial life stages are not absolute, but are epigenetic, that is, they are analogous to the Roman god Janus who had two faces, each looking in opposite directions. The individual experiencing the stage at hand is concerned with more than the present crisis. He or she is also dealing with the unfinished work of former life stages (including Basic Trust versus Basic Mistrust) and the early psychic rumblings of the period to come.

8. Pretat, *Coming to Age: The Crowning Years and Late Life Transformation*, Ch. 4. Pretat's paradigm carries Erikson's epigenetic idea a step further by suggesting that the eighth stage of Erikson's developmental theory is accompanied by the psychic resonance of several earlier states, including stage one, "Basic Trust versus Basic Mistrust."

9. Johnson, *She: Understanding Feminine Psychology.*

10. Chinen, *Once Upon a Midlife*.

11. Wheelwright, *In Old Age: The Process of Becoming an Individual*.

12. Bridges, *Transitions: Making Sense Out of Life's Changes*, p. 48. A Jungian interpretation.

13. Wheelwright, op. cit.

14. Remen, op. cit.

15. Kreinheder, *Body and Soul: The Other Side of Illness*, p. 56.

Chapter 7

1. *Holy Bible* (King James Version), Mt. 22:21–22.

2. Needleman, *Money and the Meaning of Life*, pp. 63–64.

3. Ibid, p. 72; 262–263.

4. Taylor, op. cit.

5. Frush, op. cit.

6. Frank Lloyd Wright, *An Autobiography*.

7. Gutmann, "The Cross Cultural Perspective: Notes Toward a Comparative Psychology of Aging," p. 313.

Chapter 8

1. Cumming & Henry, *Growing Old: The Process of Disengagement*. Excellent discussions of both disengagement and activity theories are found in Atchley, op. cit., and Belskey, op. cit.

2. Frush, op. cit.

3. Atchley, op. cit., p. 263.

4. Chinen, *Once Upon a Midlife*.

5. In Viorst, op. cit., p. X.

6. J. M. Macintosh, "Letter to himself."

Chapter 9

1. Lynch, *The Broken Heart*, p. 181.

2. Wolfe, *Look Homeward Angel*.

3. Hudgens, *Saints and Strangers*, p. 82.

4. In Campbell's *The Power of Myth*, p. 110.

5. John Donne, *Devotions Upon Emergent Occasions.*

6. *New Jerusalem Bible,* Gn. 7:13–16.

7. Notes from a lecture by Richard Rohr.

8. *The Jerusalem Bible,* Gn. 2:18–19.

9. Cited by Schulte, "Dying of Loneliness."

10. Ibid.

11. "Broken Heart May Trigger Alzheimer's."

12. Belsky, op. cit., p. 245.

13. Ibid.

14. An analogy suggested by Leon Epstein.

15. Belsky, op. cit., p. 240.

16. Weiss, "Loneliness."

17. *Holy Bible* (King James Version), Qo. 3:1–2.

18. Lynch, *The Language of the Heart,* p. 179.

19. Joyce, *Ulysses,* p. 32.

20. Lynch, *The Language of the Heart,* p. 146.

21. Bennet, *Meetings With Jung,* pp. 44–45.

Chapter 10

1. Hall & Lindzey, *Theories of Personality,* p. 48.

2. Russck & Schwartz, *Narrative Descriptions of Parental Love and Caring Predict Health Status in Midlife: A 35-year Follow-up of the Harvard Mastery of Stress Study,* p. 55.

3. *The Chosen,* a film directed by J. P. Kagan.

4. Viorst, op. cit., p. 73.

5. Viorst, Ibid.

6. Hollis, *The Middle Passage,* p. 11.

7. Frush, op. cit.

8. Freud, *The Future of an Illusion.*

9. Johnston, *Christian Mysticism Today,* pp. 75–76.

10. Linn & Linn, op. cit., p. 68.

11. Oxman, et al, "Lack of Social Participation or Religious Strength and Comfort as Risk Factors for Death after Cardiac Surgery in the Elderly."

12. The Rev. Richard Schmidt, Rector (Ret.), St. Paul's Episcopal Church, Daphne, Alabama.

Chapter 11

1. Wilmer, *Practical Jung: Nuts and Bolts of Jungian Psychotherapy*, p. 67.
2. Brim, *Ambition: How We Manage Success and Failure Throughout Our Lives*, p. 129.
3. Euripides, *The Trojan Women*, p. 273.
4. Behrman, *People in a Diary*, p. 115.
5. Tolstoy, *Anna Karenina*, p. 1.
6. Thoreau, *Walden*, p. 8.
7. The quotation was given to me by a friend more than twenty-five years ago. I apologize for the extent to which it is bungled.
8. St. Teresa of Avila, *Interior Castle*, p. 28.
9. Jung, "The Stages of Life," p. 17.
10. Elderhostel is a program of one-week college courses for people aged 60 and over. Hostelers live on campus or in hotels and are provided room and board. Elderhostel is a worldwide network of more than 1400 colleges and universities. Each year more than 200,000 people enroll in Elderhostel programs.

Chapter 12

1. Kennedy, *Bridging the Worlds*, Vol. 3, No. 2.
2. Chinen, *In the Ever After*.
3. Van Gennep, op. cit.
4. Vesperi, *The City of Green Benches*.
5. Adapted from Chinen, *In the Ever After*, pp. 139 ff.
6. In Bridges, op. cit., p. 44.
7. James, op. cit., p. 200.
8. Adapted from Chinen, *Once Upon a Midlife*, p. 114.
9. Ibid.
10. Wilmer, "You Zink I'm Fooling?"
11. Ibid.

Epilogue

1. Auden, "Precious Five." *Collected Shorter Poems*

1927–1957, p. 288.

2. Frost, "Dust of Snow." *The Poems of Robert Frost*, p. 233.

3. McElroy, pp. 25–26.

4. Steindl-Rast, "The Grateful Heart."

Appendix

1. Frush, op. cit., pp. 50–82.

2. See Coppersmith's *The Antecedents of Self-Esteem* and Rosenberg's *Conceiving the Self*. The instruments are, respectively, Likert (a scale with a range of choices) and Forced Choice (a scale with two choices only), and therefore amenable to scores that are quantifiable. For an exhaustive treatment of the nineteen instruments used in gerontological literature, the reader is referred to Breytspraak and George's "Self-Concept and Self-Esteem," and to Frush, op. cit., pp. 50–82.

3. Bugental, "Humanistic Psychology: A New Breakthrough." See also: Borg and Gall, *Educational Research: An Introduction* (3rd ed.); Issac and Michael, *Handbook in Research and Evaluation*; and Sellitz, Wrightsman, and Cook, *Research Methods in Social Relations* (3rd ed.).

4. Berelson, "Content Analysis," pp. 488–522; Holsti, "Content Analysis," pp. 596–692.

5. See Croog and Levine, *The Heart Patient*. Also, Croog and Levine, *Life After a Heart Attack: Social and Psychological Factors Eight Years Later*; and Rosen & Bibring, "Psychological Reactions of Hospitalized Male Patients to a Heart Attack: Age and Social-Class Differences," pp. 201–211.

References

Allport, G. (1937). *Personality: A psychological interpretation.* New York: Henry Holt.

Atchley, R. C. (1991). *Social forces and aging* (6th ed.). Belmont, CA: Wadsworth.

Auden, W. H. (1966). *Collected shorter poems 1927–1957.* New York: Random House.

Becker, E. (1973). *The denial of death.* New York: Macmillan.

Behrman, S. N. (1972). *People in a diary.* Boston: Little, Brown.

Belsky, J. K. (1990). *The psychology of aging: Theory, research, and interventions* (2nd ed.). Pacific Grove, CA: Brooks/Cole.

Bennet, E. A. (1985). *Meetings with Jung.* Zurich: Daimon.

Berelson, B. (1954). Content analysis. In G. Lindzey (Ed.), *Handbook of social psychology* (Vol. 1) (pp. 488–522). Reading, MA: Addison-Wesley.

Bly, R. (Trans.) (1983). *The Kabir book: Forty-four of the ecstatic poems of Kabir.* Boston: Beacon Hill.

Blythe, R. (1980). *The view in winter: Reflections on old age.* New York: Penguin.

Bolen, J. S. (1979). *The Tao of psychology.* San Franscisco: Harper & Row.

The book of common prayer (1977). Kingsport, TN: Kingsport.

Borg, W. R. & Gall, M. D. (1979). *Educational research: An introduction* (3rd ed.). New York: Longman.

Breytspraak, L. M., & George, L. K. (1982). Self-concept and self-esteem. In D. J. Mangen & W. A. Peterson (Eds.), *Research instruments in social gerontology: Vol. 1, Clinical and social psychology* (pp. 241–302). Minneapolis: University of Minnesota Press.

Bridges, W. (1980). *Life transitions: Making sense out of life's changes.* Reading, MA: Addison-Wesley.

Brim, O. G. (1992). *Ambition: How we manage success and failure throughout our lives.* New York: Basic Books.

Broken heart may trigger Alzheimer's. (1987, September 20). *St. Petersburg Times*.

Bugental, J. F. T. (1963). Humanistic psychology: A new breakthrough. *American Psychologist, 18*, 563–567.

Butler, R. (1975). *Why survive? Being old in America*. New York: Harper & Row.

Butterfield, S. T. (1991, May). Of lineage and love. *The Sun*, 9–15.

Campbell, J. (1985). *The power of myth*. New York: Doubleday.

Chinen, A. B. (1989). *In the ever after*. Wilmette, IL: Chiron.

Chinen, A. B. (1992). *Once upon a midlife*. Los Angeles: Tarcher.

Chopra, D. (1987). *Creating health*. Boston: Houghton Mifflin.

Clark, M. & Anderson, B. G. (1967). *Culture and aging: An anthropological study of older Americans*. Springfield, IL: Thomas.

Cooley, C. H. (1902). *Human nature and the social order*. New York: Charles Scribner's Sons.

Coppersmith, S. (1967). *The antecedents of self-esteem*. Palo Alto, CA: Consulting Psychologists Press.

Cortis, B. (1995). *Heart and soul*. New York: Villard.

Croog, S. H., & Levine, S. (1977). *The heart patient recovers*. New York: Human Sciences.

Croog, S. H., & Levine, S. (1982). *Life after a heart attack: Social and psychological factors eight years later*. New York: Human Sciences.

Cumming, E. & Henry, W. (1961). *Growing old: The process of disengagement*. New York: Basic Books.

de Beauvoir, S. (1972). *The coming of age*. P. O'Brien (Trans.). New York: Putnam.

de Tocqueville, A. (1945). *Democracy in America* Vol. II. New York: Vintage. (Original work published 1835).

Donne, J. *Devotions upon emergent occasions*, No. 17. (Original work written 1624).

Dychtwald, K. & Flower, J. (1989). *Age wave: The challenge and opportunity of an aging America*. Los Angeles: Tarcher.

Emerson, R. W. (1975). *Self Reliance*. G. Dekovic (Ed. & Photographer). New York: Funk & Wagnall's. (Original work published 1841.)

Erikson, E. H. (1963). *Childhood and society* (rev. ed.). New York: Norton.

Erikson, E. H. (1968). Generativity and ego integrity. In B. L. Neugarten (Ed.), *Middle age and aging: A reader in social psychology.* Chicago: University of Chicago Press.

Erikson, E. H., Erikson, J., & Kivnick, H. (1986). *Vital involvement in old age.* New York: Norton.

Euripides (1952). *The Trojan Women.* Chicago: Encyclopedia Britannica. (Original work first performed 5th century BCE.)

Feinstein, D. & Krippner, K. (1988). *Personal mythology.* Los Angeles: Tarcher.

Freud, L. S. (1961). The future of an illusion. In J. Strachey (Ed. & Trans.), *The standard edition of the complete psychological works of Sigmund Freud* (Vol. 21). London: Hogarts. (Original work published 1927.)

Frost, R. (1939). *The poems of Robert Frost.* New York: Modern Library.

Frush, J. (1986). *Self-esteem in older persons following a heart attack: An exploration of contributing factors.* Ann Arbor, MI: University Microfilms International.

George, L. (1993). *Financial security in later life: The subjective side.* Philadelphia: Boettner Institute of Financial Gerontology.

Gutmann, D. (1977). The cross-cultural perspective: Notes toward a comparative psychology of aging. In J. E. Birren & K. W. Schaie (Eds.), *Handbook of the psychology of aging.* New York: Van Nostrand Reinhold.

Hall, C. S., & Lindzey, G. (1978). *Theories of personality* (3rd ed.). New York: Wiley.

Hayflick, L. (1994). *How and why we age.* New York: Ballantine.

The History of Herodotus. (1952). G. Rawlinson (Trans.). Chicago: Encyclopedia Britannica. (Original work written 5th century BCE.)

Hollis, J. (1993). *The middle passage.* Toronto: Inner City.

Holsti, O. R. (1986). Content analysis. In G. Lindzey & E.

Aronson (Eds.). *The handbook of social psychology* (Vol. II) (2nd ed.) (pp. 596–692). Reading, MA: Addison-Wesley.

Holy Bible (King James Version). Camden, NJ: Nelson.

Hudgens, A. (1985). *Saints and strangers.* Boston: Houghton Mifflin.

I'Ching. (1967). R. Wilhelm (Trans.). C. F. Baynes (Trans.). Princeton, NJ: Princeton University Press.

Issac, S., & Michael, N. B. (1971). *Handbook in research and evaluation.* San Diego: Ed Its.

Jaffe, D. T. (1980). *Healing from within.* New York: Knopf.

James, W. (1952). The principles of psychology. Chicago: Encyclopedia Britannica. (Original work published 1891.)

The Jerusalem Bible (Reader's ed.). Garden City, NY: Doubleday.

John Paul II, Pope. (1986, December 9). A message to the elderly. English Edition *L'Observatore Romano,* N. 49.

Johnson, R. (1977). *She: Understanding feminine psychology.* New York: Harper & Row.

Johnson, W. (1984). *Christian mysticism today.* San Francisco: Harper & Row.

Joyce, J. (1986). *Ulysses.* New York: Random House. (Original work published 1922.)

Jung, C. G. (1965). *Memories, dreams, reflections.* (A. Jaffe, Ed.) (R. and C. Winston, Tr.). New York: Vintage.

Jung, C. G. (1976). The stages of life. In J. Campbell (Ed.), *The Portable Jung.* New York: Penguin. (Original work published 1930.)

Kagan, J. P. (Director). (1981). *The Chosen.* Film.

Keen, S. (Speaker). (1991). *Telling your story.* Cassette. New York: Sound Horizons.

Keen, S. & Moyers, B. *Your mythic journey.* Film.

Kennedy, A. *Bridging the worlds,* 3 (2). Soquel, CA: Author.

Kopp, S. B. (1972). *If you meet the Buddha on the road, kill him!* New York: Bantam.

Kreinheder, A. (1991). *Body and soul: The other side of illness.* Toronto: Inner City.

Levin, W. C. (1994). Age stereotyping: College student evaluations. *Aging* (9th ed.). Guilford, CT: Dushkin.

Lewis, R. (1994, February). For whom the job bell doesn't toll. *AARP Bulletin.*

Linn, D. & Linn, M. (1978). *Healing life's hurts: Healing memories through the five stages of forgiveness.* New York: Paulist.

Lynch, James J. (1977). *The broken heart.* New York: Basic Books.

Lynch, James J. (1985). *The language of the heart.* New York: Basic Books.

Macintosh, J. M. (1956). Letter to himself. Personal papers. *The Lancet,* 809–810.

May, R. (1991). *The cry for myth.* New York: Norton.

McElroy, S. C. (1996). *Animals as teachers and healers.* New York: Ballantine.

McDougall, W. (1935). *The energies of men.* (3rd ed.). London: Methuen.

McLean, C. (1994). The graying of America. *Aging* (9th ed.). Guilford, CT: Dushkin.

Melamed, E. (1983). *Mirror, mirror: The terror of not being young.* New York: Linden.

Miller, A. (1949). *Death of a salesman.* New York: Viking.

Mobile Register (1994, May 13). Middle-aged men risk layoffs.

Mobile Register (1994, July 4). Job bias complaints swamp investigators.

Needleman, J. (1991). *Money and the meaning of life.* New York: Doubleday.

Neugarten, B. L. (1977). Personality and aging. In J. E. Birren & K. W. Schaie (Eds.), *Handbook of the psychology of aging.* New York: Van Nostrand Reinhold.

O'Bryant, S. L. (1991). Older widows and independent life styles. *The International Journal of Aging and Human Development,* 32, (1), 41–51.

Oregon to fund assisted suicide for poor. (1999, January). *Housing for the Elderly Report.* Silver Springs, MD: CD.

Oxman, T. E., et al. (1995). Lack of social participation or religious strength and comfort as risk factors for death after cardiac surgery in the elderly. *Psychosomatic Medicine,* 57,

681–689.

Palmore, E. (1970). Normal aging. *Reports from the Duke Longitudinal Study, 1955–1969.* Durham, NC: Duke University Press.

Palmore, E. (1974). Normal Aging II. *Reports from the Duke Longitudinal Study, 1970–1973.* Durham, NC: Duke University Press.

Pascal, B. (1952). *Pensees.* W. F. Trotter (Trans.). Chicago: Encyclopedia Britannica. (Original work published 1670.)

Percy, W. (1981). *Lanterns on the levee.* Baton Rouge, LA: Louisiana State University Press. (Original work published 1941.)

Pretat, J. R. (1994). *Coming to age: The croning years and late-life transformation.* Toronto: Inner City.

Remen, R. N. (Speaker). *The eye of an eagle, the heart of a lion, the hand of a woman.* Cassette recording NMT 140. Berkeley: New Medicine Tapes.

Rohr, R. (1993, January). Paper presented at St. Pius X Catholic Church, Mobile, AL.

Rosen, J. L., & Bibring, G. L. (1968). Psychological reactions of hospitalized male patients to a heart attack: Age and social class differences. In B. L. Neugarten (Ed.), *Middle age and aging: a reader in social psychology* (pp. 201–211). Chicago: University of Chicago Press.

Rosenberg, M. (1965). *Society and the adolescent self-image.* Princeton, N.J.: Princeton University Press.

Rosenberg, M. (1979). *Conceiving the self.* New York: Basic Books.

Russek, L. G., & Schwartz, G. E. (1996). Narrative descriptions of parental love and caring predict health status in midlife: A 35-year follow-up of the Harvard Mastery of Stress Study. *Alternative Therapies,* 4 (6), 55–62.

St. Teresa of Avila (1961). *Interior castle.* E. A. Peers (Trans). New York: Doubleday. (Original work written 1577.)

Schulte, J. (1987, September 20). Dying of loneliness. *St. Petersburg Times.*

Seligman, M. E. P. (1991). *Learned optimism*. New York: Knopf.

Sellitz, C., Wrightsman, L. S., & Cook, S. W. (1976). *Research methods in social relations* (3rd ed.). New York: Holt, Rinehart & Winston.

Shakespeare, W. (1952). *Hamlet*. Chicago: Encyclopedia Britannica (Original work performed 1600–1601.)

Shakespeare, W. (1952). *King Lear*. Chicago: Encyclopedia Britannica (Original work performed 1605–1606.)

Skinner, B. F. & Vaughan, M. E. (1983). *Enjoy old age: A program of self-management*. New York: Norton.

Staff. (1944, May). More on anger and heart disease. *Harvard Heart Letter*, (7)9 , p. 7.

Stein, M. (1981). *In midlife*. Dallas: Spring.

Steindl-Rast, D. (Speaker). (1992). *The grateful heart*. Cassette recording. Boulder, CO: Sounds True.

Stevens, K. (Host). *Life in prime time*. Film.

Swift, J. (1952). *Gulliver's Travels*. Chicago: Encyclopedia Britannica. (Original work published 1726.)

Taylor, S. E. (1983). Adjustment to threatening events: A theory of cognitive adaptation. *American Psychologist*, 38, (11), 1161–1173.

Thoreau, H. D. (1973). *Walden*. Princeton, NJ: Princeton University Press. (Original work published 1854.)

Tolstoy, L. (1952). *Anna Karenina*. Chicago: Encyclopedia Britannica. (Original work published 1877.)

van Gennep, A. (1960). *The rite of passage*. M. B. Vizedom & G.L. Caffee (Trans.). London: Routledge & Kegan Paul. (Original work published 1909.)

Vesperi, M. (1985). *The city of green benches*. Ithaca, NY: Cornell University Press.

Viorst, J. (1987). *Necessary losses*. New York: Fawcett.

Weiss, R. S. (1988, June). Loneliness. *The Harvard Medical School Mental Health Letter*, 4 (12) p. 5.

Wheelwright, J. (Speaker) (1988). *In old age: The process of becoming an individual*. Cassette recording. San Francisco: C. G. Jung Institute.

Wilmer, H. A. (1987). *Practical Jung: Nuts and bolts of Jungian psychotherapy*. Wilmette, IL: Chiron.

Wilmer, H. A. (Speaker) (1990). "You zink I'm fooling?" Cassette recording. San Francisco: C. G. Jung Institute.

Winklevoss, H. E. & Powell, A. V. (1984). *Continuing care retirement communities: An empirical, financial, and legal analysis*. Homewood, IL: Richard D. Irwin.

Wolfe, T. (1929). *Look homeward angel*. New York: Scribners.

Wright, F. L. (1943). *An autobiography*. New York: Duell, Sloan, and Pearce.

Yalom, I. D. (1989). *Love's executioner and other tales of psychotherapy*. New York: Harper Collins.

Yeats, W. B. (1958). The coming of wisdom with time. *Collected Poems*. New York: Macmillan. (Original work published 1910.)

Index

activity theory and,
105
partial, 105–11
resistance to, 105
smooth, 104
theory of, 104
Donne, John, 115
Doppelgangers, 64–74
defined, 64–65
negative, 72–74
personal myth and,
65–71
Dormoy, Marie, 70–71
Dreams, 148, 155
Dying young, 15–16

"Eating your heart out,"
78–80
Ecclesiastes, 20, 120
Ego integrity, 42–43
Einstein, Albert, 146
Elderhostel, 145
"Elder tales," 147
see also Fairy tales
Elizabethan theater, 22–23
Elusinian mysteries, 89–90
Embarrassment, 64
Emerson, Ralph Waldo, 86
Emptiness, 71
Epictetus, 33
Epstein, Leon, 117–18
Erikson, Erik, 42, 76, 88
Erikson, Joan, 76
Eros, 90–92
Euripides, 138
Explanatory style, 59–63

Fairy tales, 146–61
about older persons,
146–49
about young people,
146, 147–48
coming to terms
with one's lot
and, 155–57
consciousness and,
153, 154
defined, 146
detours and, 158–59
dreams and, 148,
155
liminal state and,
148–49, 153
mercurial quality,
154–55
money and, 149–55

"Shining Fish,"
149–55
"Stonecutter,"
156–57
as teaching stories,
147
Fathers, 124–35
afterthought,
134–35
Bible and, 126
daughters and, 126
father hunger,
127–28
heart attack sur-
vivors and,
129–34
perceptions of God
and, 130–32
religion and,
132–35
sons and, 126–27,
128–29
Faulkner, William, 85
Fear:
of death, 133–34
of lack of money,
95–102
of loss of self-
reliance,
85–89
Fisher, M. F. K., 136
Fitzgerald, F. Scott, 95
Foolishness, 146–61
Forgetfulness, 80
Forgiveness, 79, 80–81
Fortune, 53
Franciscan order, 122
Frankfurter, Felix, 140
Freud, Sigmund, 124, 131,
134
Frost, Robert, 165
Functional impairment, 25

Gandhi, 42
Garbo, Greta, 138
Gardening, 107–108
Generativity, 88–89
fairy tales and, 154
Genesis, 115
"George," 48, 127–28
Geriatrics, 72
Gerontological Society of
America,
103–104
God, 94
Caesar and, 98, 99,

102
fairy tales and, 154
fathers and percep-
tions of,
130–32,
134–35
loneliness and,
115–16, 123
Grace, 46, 158
Grapes of Wrath, The
(Steinbeck),
32
Great Depression, 87
Greek mythology, 76, 78
celebration of har-
vest, 89–90
"going home" sto-
ries, 92–93
memory and, 80
synchronicity, 52–53
trust and, 90–92
Grief, stages of, 81–83
Grotjahn, M., 23
Gulliver's Travels (Swift),
23, 164
Gutmann, David, 101–102

Hades, 52, 89
Hamlet (Shakespeare), 22
Harte, Brett, 45
Harvard Mastery of Stress
Study, 125
Health care reform, 18–19
Heart attack survivors, 27
causes of heart
attacks, 61–62
disengagement and,
107–10
fathers and, 129–34
money and, 96–102
research methodolo-
gy, 167–70
self-affirmation of,
100–101
self-esteem of, 38,
47, 53, 60–62
Heart disease, 79–80
loneliness and, 116
Heart surgery, 162–66
Hector, 52
Heifetz, Jascha, 58–59
Helen of Troy, 93
Helplessness, 60
Hermes, 52–53
Hero and the Goddess,
The

Kind Hearts

Kind Hearts